Your Choice

Becoming Empowered to Participate in Your Own Health Care

2nd Edition

Hernán Drobny, MD

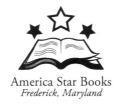

America Star Books
Frederick, Maryland

Hardcover 9781683943662
Softcover 9781683943655
eBook 9781630848187
PUBLISHED BY AMERICA STAR BOOKS, LLLP
www.americastarbooks.pub
Frederick, Maryland

To Ann

Words are not necessary or sufficient

Proceeds from this book
will be dedicated to improve
the health and well-being of people
whose difficulties came about through
no choice of their own

There but for fortune, may go you or I

Phil Ochs

Table of Contents

Acknowledgments...9
Preface...11
Prologue 17

Section 1—How We Make Health Care Decisions.....................25
Chapter 1—Exercising Autonomy in Medical Decision Making.....29
Chapter 2—Perceptions of Risk..36
Chapter 3—Emotions and Bias..44

Section 2—The Process...55
Chapter 4—Going to the Doctor..59
Chapter 5—More Care is not Necessarily Better Care.....................68
Chapter 6—Thieves of Autonomy 82

Section 3—Aging and Health Care 89
Chapter 7—Aging and Health Care Choices—Preparing to go Slow 93
Chapter 8—Choices as the End of Life Approaches 108
Chapter 9—Advance Directives 123

Section 4—Planning and Clarifying.................................135
Chapter 10—Gathering Information...................................139
Chapter 11—Participation in Clinical Research 153
Chapter 12—Health Care Teams: The Importance of Experience and
    Volume 160

Section 5—Personal Observations and Perspectives................169
Personal Observation 1—The Forest and the Trees: Treating the
    Numbers or Treating the Patient 173
Personal Observation 2—Expectations...................................176
Personal Observation 3—Support: Often a Help, Sometimes a
    Hindrance 179
Personal Observation 4—Caregivers Need Support Too.................183
Personal Observation 5—Choosing a Primary Care Physician 186

Epilogue 194
Supplementary Material....................................199
References...224
Index 241

Acknowledgments

A comment at a chance encounter on the street, a story told at a social gathering, a question asked at a forum, a concern expressed in the locker-room, an anecdote described while looking for a golf ball, a thought revealed at a community event: so many people contributed ideas for this book. I appreciate your willingness to share experiences, and I hope that this book will prove useful as a result. I am sorry that not all of the seeds you offered survived as material for this project.

I am grateful to my patients over the years: for opening your hearts and lives, and having the confidence to share your intimate concerns with me, and allowing me to participate in your health care. Your experiences and stories form the backbone of this book.

My parents, Abraham and Gladys Drobny, always provided support and encouragement (as well as other means parents use to influence their children), in my endeavors, this book included. Muchisimas gracias, siempre.

David Scarrat, PhD, scientist, editor, and friend found ways to improve the clarity of the material by using less but more effective words. You are a "wordsmith"; thanks again.
David Share, MD, colleague, and friend, thanks for your wise and caring comments on the manuscript and helping me separate my opinions from evidence.

My wife, Ann Barden, to whom this book is dedicated, was with me from the first seed that led to the suggestion that this project could end up as a book, to the last period on the last page. Always believing I could complete this project, sometimes in front pulling, sometimes behind me pushing, but mostly by my side supporting, advising, and improving the material: this book would not exist without you. Thanks for everything.

Preface
Your Health, Your Choice

Health care today presents many choices. We choose the type of health care provider to consult. We may need to decide which tests are the best ones to use for diagnosing and managing a health condition, or be faced with choices of what treatments, medications, and procedures might be best for each particular situation. The central theme of this book is your right to participate in making those choices: **the exercise of individual autonomy in health care**. My premise is that actively participating in making health care decisions, and taking responsibility for these decisions, improves your health care outcomes and your quality of life, as well as lowering the cost of health care. Active participation in making health care decisions is often referred to as making an "**informed choice**".

A fundamental principle of medical ethics is respect for patient autonomy. The physician is guided by the principle of respecting your right to make personal decisions about matters affecting your health. To exercise this right, you need to understand the options and be able to express your choice among them clearly and effectively.

This not a simple or easy process, however.

Medical decisions can be complicated and overwhelming, and choices may have to be made under duress. Perhaps you may be feeling unwell and afraid. At these times it is difficult to think clearly and critically. Often there are no easy answers, and it seems simpler to have others choose for you.

As the medical system has become more complex and specialized, it has become increasingly difficult to obtain objective information without conflicts of interest or bias. You need this kind of information in order to make wise choices. It has also become more complicated to navigate the health care delivery system and to obtain the consultations and information necessary to make an informed choice. In this book I explore issues such as:

- How you benefit from participating in making personal medical decisions.
- How emotions, beliefs, and irrational reactions influence the choices you make.
- How your understanding and view of risk can affect your decisions.
- How to prepare to go to the doctor so that all your concerns will be considered.
- How to obtain reliable medical information.
- How to avoid the tendency to use more medical treatments, procedures, and technologies than are necessary.
- Why you sometimes surrender your autonomy.
- How you can best ensure that your wishes regarding health care choices will be carried out if you're not capable of expressing them due to a physical or mental inability (through legal documents called "Advance Directives").
- How advanced age may influence your health care choices.
- How to consider the option of participating in clinical investigations.
- Where you should go to obtain the services you need.
- How to choose a primary care provider.
- Why having personal support can improve the ability to make good choices.

A New Medical Specialty

During my years of clinical practice my interest in how patients make medical decisions grew. I wanted my patients to understand their medical conditions and to discuss the choices available for diagnosing and managing them. I saw that it was necessary to allow space and time for that person to make a decision. I began to read and discuss decision making from an academic perspective and to see if I could integrate some of this knowledge into the practical realm of working with patients. Of course, clearly defined topics in academia became less clear cut in the practical world. There were issues that could not be pigeon-holed into one category. Sometimes, personal situations influenced the reactions to the medical concerns, perhaps creating contradictions when making a critically considered choice. Yet having a conceptual structure from which to start was helpful in analyzing the situation.

After 32 years in primary care practice in Internal Medicine at the University of Michigan, I established a consulting practice as a patient advocate, with the purpose of promoting individual autonomy in health care decisions. I researched and studied the academic information on decision making and participated in the Decision Making Consortium of the University of Michigan. In this new area of work, I have consulted with individuals who wanted help with medical concerns. They sometimes needed help in navigating the medical establishment, or even in deciding what kind of help would be most useful. At other times, I have worked with individuals who need to make an important medical decision, and who wanted someone with no conflicts of interest to help them consider what to do. For example, a coronary bypass was recommended to a patient by a cardiac surgeon, but a cardiologist did not agree that it was necessary. An invasive test, like an arteriogram, was suggested to evaluate an aneurysm (a blood vessel weakness) by a radiologist who performs these tests; was this the best approach to assess this problem or is there a less invasive test? Commonly, after a cancer diagnosis, the choice of what is the best treatment or management causes much confusion. Sometimes there was an uncertainty in the diagnosis and the question of what steps might clarify it needed to be addressed.

"Oh, great," you may be thinking, "not another type of specialty in medical care." The irony is that medicine has become so specialized and fragmented, with liver, kidney, nervous system, heart, skin, bone, diabetes, blood, and so many other specialists who have very focused views. A specialty that can provide a bridge to connect the various concerns, that can provide broader and more comprehensive perspective on the whole person and their personal values and preferences, can be helpful. It is a specialty that can coordinate among the different specialties and health care providers, and a specialty that can advocate for the individual and his or her family. This could be done by the primary care provider or family doctor, but today these doctors are often too busy, and many people don't have a primary care provider.

Making Medical Decisions

Daniel Kahneman won the Nobel Prize in Economics in 2002 for his work over 30 years in decision making under conditions of uncertainty. Medical decisions, too, are made under conditions of uncertainty. The study of decision making has now become a growing area of study and research in universities. Some of these concepts are being applied to medical decision making. Work has been concentrated on the ways doctors make decisions, but information on how patients make decisions is increasing.

I strive, in this book, to offer some practical approaches and perspectives for you to be an effective participant in making medical decisions, and to feel empowered in advocating for yourself and your family. My goal is to help you and those you care about to get the best medical care. This is best accomplished by becoming an effective and active participant in health care decisions. I want you to understand how people commonly make decisions about their health care. What are the pitfalls? How might these pitfalls be avoided? I provide a framework to help you prepare before visiting a health care provider. There are suggestions on how to increase your understanding of the plan for your medical care so that you are more likely to follow that plan. There are questions you may want to ask prior to having diagnostic tests or treatments. I offer some ways of thinking about particular situations so that you can make wise choices, such as whether to participate in research trials or how to choose a decision maker for you in a situation where you cannot make the decision yourself.

This book is organized into several sections. One section, "*How We Make Health Care Decisions*" describes some of the benefits of "informed choice", as well as some pitfalls in making decisions. "*The Process*" talks about interacting with your doctors and health care providers. It offers tools and ideas that help assure that you will get your health care needs met with quality and completeness. "*Aging and Health Care Choices" focuses* on the influence that advancing age may have on the choices you make. "*Planning and Clarifying*" provides ways of thinking about particular issues in advance, and how to obtain information to prepare you to make decisions carefully. In the section titled "*Personal Observations*", I offer a perspective based on my experiences in particular topics that seem relevant and are connected to many of the topics I cover in this book. The *Supplementary Material* offers further information that is relevant to the topics in the book and can help you understand the medical system. In the *References*, I provide references to books and articles from which I derive many of the facts and ideas mentioned in the text. The chapters can be read in sequence, or you can pick and choose the sections and chapters that suit your current needs and situations.

To simplify the text, I may use either him or her when both may be appropriate. The cases that illustrate concepts presented in the book are based on real experiences. The names of the patients have been changed to minimize any intrusion into their privacy.

Prologue

It has been my belief that having patients participate in making informed choices in partnership with their health care providers, supports the practice of high-quality medicine. I came to this position gradually through my experiences as a primary care physician. Now, I find it supported by a growing body of information in the medical literature. Seeing how I came to this view from the perspective of a health care provider provides another way for health care consumers to understand why this partnership and joint decision making are necessary to ensure the provision of comprehensive and high-quality medical care.

My desire to become a doctor was in part based on idealism and a hope for the good I could do as a "healer". During my medical school years at the University of Pennsylvania and post-graduate training in Michigan during the 1970s, my focus was on mastering the ever-expanding body of scientific knowledge. I was afraid of not knowing the crucial piece of information that would cause my patient to suffer or die. It was and is necessary to stay current with new developments in medicine. My idealism was suspended.

During our training, discussion of the complexities and intricacies of the professional relationship between physicians and their patients was not carefully examined. There was little or no discussion of the importance of that relationship. Professors assumed since we were budding professionals, that we had knowledge and understanding of medical ethics.

The Real World

Early in my experience in the "real world" of medical practice, I grudgingly learned that my desire to apply all of the scientific principles and knowledge I had acquired was not possible without some negotiation, discussion, and "buy-in" from the patient. Patients often had legitimate questions that my scientific training had not prepared me to answer. As my experience grew, I found it stimulating to have a frank discussion with my patients about the options available. It was common for the patient to offer a perspective as we talked that I had not considered, giving me an opportunity to learn from them. Engaging with a patient in a discussion of their conditions encouraged me to look for good articles and information on their choices. I saw my ability to share information and honestly offer the various approaches based on medical evidence grow. I saw that without a "buy-in" and without a clear understanding of the medical plan to diagnose and treat a condition, the patient was less likely to adhere to the plan, regardless of the scientific evidence supporting it.

In the early days of my practice, a senior officer of the University came to see me with a scratchy throat. I evaluated him and told him this was an early viral infection and gave him some ideas for self-care to help him feel better. He said, "I want penicillin. It always nips these viruses as they are starting. I have an important meeting in the morning." I told him that penicillin was for bacterial infections, and it had no effect on viruses, and could cause adverse effects. He was adamant and so was I! He left angry, went to the director of our clinic to complain, and was given a prescription for penicillin. I was given a compassionate lecture on science versus belief in the practice of medicine. "A strong belief, be it in religion or medicine is difficult to argue with. Sometimes it is best not to even try," I was told.

Strong opinions (based on their training, experiences, and beliefs) are frequently offered by different specialists for options in diagnosing and treating medical conditions. In cases of prostate cancer, for example, surgeons specializing in urology often feel strongly that surgery offers the best hope for a cure. Medical oncologists feel that some of these men would do better with chemotherapy. Radiation oncologists think that many of these men would have better results by using radiation treatment as part of the approach. There are alternative and complementary health care providers who feel a dietary approach is best. Each of these specialists believes in what they are offering and can offer evidence to support their opinion. They have the best of intentions, but each also stands to gain from promoting the option they offer. Beliefs can become so strongly felt that they are confused to be facts.

Over time, I saw more and more conflicts of this type. There are doctors who recommend a test or procedure that they or a staff member will perform in their office. This can be a cardiologist suggesting an exercise test or a gastroenterologist recommending a colonoscopy or a dermatologist offering to freeze a skin blemish for example. Sometimes the indications for these procedures or tests are not entirely clear to me. It is a built-in conflict of interest in the way medicine is practiced in many parts of the world. It is a subtle bias but does have influence in the recommendations that medical practitioners make. I am not referring to the obvious commercialism of promoting unproven tests and treatments, like body scans or health spas treating cancers with an expensive unproven therapy. I am referring to proven tests and treatments with risks and benefits that need to be carefully weighed. I found that a shared participation in these considerations with my patients broadened their perspective of their choices. I could, therefore, share the responsibilities for weighing with my patients their options for each situation. This made the separation of opinions from evidence clearer.

More than one approach may be suitable for a given situation. Depending on your values, preferences, and life station, completely different choices might be reasonable for the management of the same medical problem. A person who travels as part of their work may choose a treatment that requires less monitoring and observation than someone who stays in one location most of the time. So if a person has an enlarged lymph gland, for example, she may choose to observe it over several months prior to doing a biopsy because the biopsy may not be necessary if the lymph node gets smaller. Another reasonable choice could be to remove it and obtain a definitive diagnosis in order to avoid the need for continued monitoring. Some patients may find that anxiety intrudes in their life, by always thinking about the possible problems that the enlarged lymph node may indicate. For them, removing it earlier may be the wise choice.

An example of this was when Roland came to see me late one afternoon with a very sore throat and a fever that had started 2 days before. His urgency was that he was leaving for Morocco in the morning. After evaluating him, I said that he had about a 20% chance that it was strep throat, a bacterial infection, but more likely it was a viral infection. Normally, we would prefer to do a culture and only treat with antibiotics if it is positive the next day. This prevents the 3-5% chance of side effects from the drug, as well as the concern of overusing antibiotics. But he was leaving early the following morning and could not get his results easily. He preferred to risk the side effects of taking antibiotics, even if not necessary, to not treating the 20% probability of a bacterial infection. We both understood that if he was not traveling the next day, the choice of treatment would have been different. Medical science and evidence can only go so far. Different situations and values, different emotional concerns, different resources, competing work or life responsibilities, all call for differing approaches.

Carol presented another type of situation: she came to see me with diarrhea, nausea, and fever. After the evaluation, I described the different possible approaches for testing and treating her condition. She said, "Doctor, I feel terrible. Just tell me what to do to get better." She was not very interested in weighing options or discussing the risks and benefits of the various treatment possibilities.

The relationship between a health care provider and a patient is a unique one in our society. It must be recognized that the state of being ill can make an individual lose their confidence, to regress and be more childlike. The doctor has power and influence due to his special knowledge and position. You share intimate information with your doctors, facts, and feelings you may not share with anyone else. This must be respected.

Medical Ethics

As I've stated, when I was a medical student, there was not much discussion of medical ethics and professionalism. In my years of practice, though, I have found that referring to some basic principles of medical ethics has supported making skillful decisions in difficult situations. Truly following medical ethical principles is not just being virtuous or "doing the right thing". It actually leads to better outcomes for individuals and for society.

There are four fundamental principles of medical ethics. These basic principles are not mutually exclusive or absolute, but must be balanced by health care providers. **Autonomy** is the principle that states that individuals have the right to choose the medical care they prefer, but that the choices made must be within the confines of the other basic principles. Sometimes, however, patients are not prepared to participate in making choices for their medical care. **Beneficence** means that the best interests of the individual patient a physician is attending must be foremost. **Non-maleficence** means a doctor must do their best to see that no harm comes to that individual as a result of their medical care. **Justice** is the one principle that applies to society at large, not just to the individual in front of the physician. The choices made for that individual must be balanced with the effect they may have on the rest of society.

One example: is screening for cancer in the best interest of the individual or might it be harmful? We can cause harm by overdoing medical care, by not intervening and testing enough, or by misusing medical testing and treatment. It clearly is possible to harm a patient by testing and treating a prostate cancer or a breast cancer if that cancer was never going to harm him. Some cancers are "innocent" in that they grow very slowly or not at all. A man over 75 years old with a prostate cancer is more likely to die *with* the cancer (due to some other process, perhaps a heart problem) than *from* the cancer. On the other hand, some prostate cancers may spread and cause pain and death, particularly in younger men. So far we have not been very precise in knowing which men will benefit from treating their prostate cancers, or which cancers will never cause harm, and which cancers are too late to benefit from treatment once they are discovered. The costs of screening and treatments are borne by society at large as well as the individual patients and their families. The balancing act of these principles is continuous and sometimes complex. Since we are dealing with uncertainty, it is understood that all tests, procedures, and treatments may have benefits and risks and costs.

A Personal and Illustrative Anecdote

I remember when Professor Nwango, a Nigerian man in his early 60s arrived at my office with a gift. He told me he was thanking me for saving his life! 8 weeks prior to this visit he had had an operation to remove his prostate gland called a radical prostatectomy because he was found to have cancer within it. It was thought to be an early cancer and he was told that the surgery was successful in removing the entire tumor. He felt very optimistic. Since his operation, he was having urinary incontinence, but he was confident this would soon lessen. And even if he would end up with continued difficulty with erections, which is common after this surgery, he would still be alive, working, and spending time with his family.

6 months prior to this visit he had come for a physical exam. During this exam, I had found a slight irregularity in his prostate. When I told him of this, he was worried and asked what he should do. I offered several possible approaches, but he really wanted me to tell him what to do. And it was clear that he wanted to do *something*. So we proceeded to the next step, getting a blood test for the PSA (prostate-specific antigen) level which is sometimes elevated with prostate abnormalities, including cancer. His was moderately high, above the normal level.

Again, what to do? Doing something was necessary for him. "Watchful waiting", which involves periodic testing and reevaluation was not enough. He was scheduled for a biopsy which proved positive for cancer, and which in turn led to the surgery to remove his prostate. And now, he was so grateful that I had saved his life. I know I had not *saved* his life, but finding the cancer may possibly have *prolonged* it.

Treatment for prostate cancer is controversial. Some studies appear to suggest that treatment may modestly prolong a patient's life, while others show no benefit of treatment. Most of the time, finding cancer leads to some form of treatment, most commonly surgery or radiation therapy, but it is clear that treatment causes some harm. There are also other costs of treatment, including financial costs, lost time from work, and feeling poorly for a time, as well as urinary incontinence and difficulties with erections.

The issues around prostate cancer screening and treatment are complex. In part, this is due to the lack of definitive evidence that screening for cancers make people live longer, that it saves lives. Screening for colon cancer for those at elevated risk for developing one, for example, does decrease the chances of dying from those cancers because early detection of a pre-cancerous growth can lower the risk of developing cancer or it can lead to effective treatments. This has not yet been shown to be the case in prostate cancer. But there is also a lot of emotion around cancer, including those arising in the prostate. Many health care professionals have strong opinions on what is the right thing to do when it is diagnosed. These opinions are as diverse as differences we have in politics, spiritual beliefs, and who is the best basketball player.

Helping a man and his family really understand these issues takes time and effort, time that is often not available in a busy medical practice. It is more efficient for the clinician to say, "I think we should get a blood test to see if you may have a cancer of the prostate." There is the sense you are taking care of him, that you are looking out for his best interests, and legally, that you are not taking the risk of being negligent in his care.

Professor Nwango's gratitude made me feel ill at ease. Perhaps I had only participated in making him incontinent and leaving him with sexual dysfunction. He had not wanted to make the decision himself, yet in a way he had decided that he wanted to do something after the slight abnormality was brought to his attention. But, maybe I should never even have examined his prostate without first informing him that if an abnormality was detected it could ultimately lead to a diagnosis which could result in an invasive procedure as a treatment, which could result in incontinence and impotence.

The idea of patients being autonomous and participating fully in informed decision making in their medical care is not universal. Professor Nwango had been teaching at a large university in the U.S. for six years. In Africa and elsewhere in the world, a more paternalistic and autocratic style of medical practice is more common than that in the U.S. and Western Europe. In my experience in the practice of medicine over the last three decades, patients have become increasingly involved in making decisions that affect their own medical care. But people of different generations and different cultural backgrounds react differently to this concept.

I have seen in my clinical experience in Mexico and in my travels in South America and Asia that participation in making health care choices by individual patients and their families is unusual. Sometimes frank information about a medical condition is kept from the patient and the rest of the family as a way of protecting them from fears that the information may elicit. Yet I also saw great appreciation when time and effort were taken in helping patients understand as much as possible about their medical problems.

More research on the influences affecting decision making is regularly being reported. There is a growing acceptance that collaborative decision making between the patients and their families and their health care providers improves the outcomes and benefits individuals and society. This manuscript is an attempt to share my experience and my conceptual framework in the hope that it may be useful to you.

Section 1

How We Make Health Care Decisions

There is evidence revealing that there are benefits in being involved in making your own medical decisions. However, to be able to make wise health care decisions, there are a number of factors to consider. This section is about the *process* of making health care decisions by the individual affected directly by the choices.

As my interest in decision making by patients developed, I found that the subject has become a growing field in the academic world. Colleagues in business and marketing, public health, public policy, political science, economics, psychology, as well as in medicine are specializing and doing research in this.

In medicine, much of the interest has been in how doctors reach their decisions. Now there is new interest and work being done on how patients reach decisions. There has been growth in understanding that there are patterns and influences in how people make decisions in everyday life, including how we make decisions regarding our health care.

The study of this area has revealed that we often take shortcuts in making decisions, and therefore miss opportunities to fully weigh all the factors and possible consequences. We all have built-in prejudices that can bias our decisions, even though we may be unaware of these influences in this process. This section shows how the "shortcuts" can cause you to make decisions without fully reviewing the consequences and benefits of all the options. Also, your own personal patterns of how you categorize risk may inadvertently influence the decisions you make. When you become more aware of these patterns and understand their influences, you can avoid some hazards and pitfalls. As a result, you can make better, more critically considered decisions.

Chapter 1

Exercising Autonomy in Medical Decision Making

It is important and desirable that individuals participate actively in making medical decisions, and take responsibility for them.

A **fundamental principle of medical ethics** is that patients are autonomous and therefore have the **right of choice** in their medical care. Physicians are obligated to support this right. This is often referred to as **informed choice.**

Individuals have a **legal right** to make personal medical choices. This legal right is called *informed consent*. Specifically, patients have a legal right to agree to or reject diagnostic and treatment recommendations, and that this consent must be based on an understanding of adequate and accurate information.

These ethical and legal rights also bring benefits. Patients have a greater and clearer understanding of the choices they make and are more likely to follow their treatment plans if they participated in making the choices. Studies have shown that people have greater satisfaction with their medical care when they participate in making the decisions for their care.

There is empirical evidence from studies comparing "usual care" and informed choice. In these studies, some patients were given the opportunity to make decisions after a thorough discussion of the information and choices available for diagnosis and treatment. Other patients were provided the information in a more traditional (paternalistic) style. Comparison of the two groups showed that the active involvement of individuals in making their medical decisions led to better outcomes.

- Satisfaction with care and adherence with medical programs is enhanced.
- Patients express greater confidence in their health care and the recommendations made.
- Psychological adjustment to illness is improved.
- There is a greater resolution of symptoms.
- Control of chronic conditions, like diabetes and hypertension, is improved.
- Psychological well-being is improved.
- Individuals making their own decisions choose fewer prescriptions, and as a result take less medicine.
- Fewer individuals making their own decisions choose to have surgical procedures.
- The overall costs of health care are lower.
- There is no loss in quality of life or health due to patient involvement in making medical decisions for themselves or their family members.

Better results with fewer interventions and fewer medications at a lower cost. That is the **good news**!

The bad news is that health care, as it is currently practiced, is not usually structured to help patients make informed decisions regarding their health care. According to a published review, informed decision making, where patients are given evidence and options and are asked to participate, occurred in only 9% of outpatient visits. *In fewer than half of the doctor visits did the physician ask if the patient had any questions about what was discussed or advised.*

Patients sometimes do not want to make decisions. Understanding the information and the probabilities of benefits and harms can be difficult. They may be afraid of making a bad choice, and making wise decisions may seem beyond their ability. The process of making decisions and taking responsibility for decisions that have substantial risks and uncertain outcomes may be emotionally daunting.

The ideal process in making a complex decision involves gathering information and calculating the benefits and costs of each option. The optimal choice is then reached by a careful review of this evidence and these calculations. Benjamin Franklin was an early pioneer in this "decision analysis". He followed a simple approach of listing all the positives of each option in one column and the negatives in another. He would cross out each of the listed benefits in column A that equaled a cost in column B. He then would see what was left in each column. The option with most positives or fewest negatives would be his choice.

However, patients usually reach judgments using their intuition or base their choice on greatly simplified logic and limited information. Sometimes the decisions are influenced by what family members or friends have done in similar situations, relying more on what is familiar to them than an informed choice based on information and judgment. The decision making process is frequently affected by emotions and fears. We take mental shortcuts, which increase the chances of misperceptions and bias. These shortcuts are referred to as **heuristics** in the field of decision making.

In much of everyday life, the use of heuristics seems to work out reasonably well. It can save time and worry. There are situations, however, when you should avoid shortcuts. A different process is called for if the decision has long-term consequences or has possible risks that are considered "major". In these circumstances, you need to avoid bias as well as understand the risks involved. This process must be as clear as possible for you to reach a wise decision.

I see four necessary factors in making a sound medical decision:

- Gathering information.
- Understanding the information, and being clear about potential risks and benefits.
- Taking time to consider the information and the options available, keeping in mind the likely nature of the experience which will be associated with the different options.

• Considering personal preferences and values in the context of this information.

Gathering **reliable information** is a complex task which we'll discuss in more detail in chapter 10. In addition to reviewing the medical literature, looking at medical texts, and considering the information provided by the consulting doctors, there are thousands of websites in many languages discussing health care on the internet. An internet search for "health care" (defined as the prevention, treatment, and management of illness and the preservation of mental and physical well-being through the services offered by the medical and allied health professions) using the Google search engine, yielded more than 900 million hits. A Harvard group specializing in medical information on the internet concluded that more than *95% of these are suspect*. They may be compromised by conflicts of interest, such as when the site is associated with the sale of products or services. On other sites, the information and recommendations were based on beliefs that are justified by pseudoscience (for further discussions on "pseudoscience" refer to Chapter 10, *Gathering Information*).

A chilling view of the internet era warns that high-quality information will be overwhelmed by low-quality information. This is because the cost of producing and maintaining web portals with lower quality of information is much less than that of websites of higher quality. In order to assure that quality standards are met, expert authorities must assess the quality of the information before it is posted on the internet, which requires funding. The cost of distributing the information, however, is the same and very small whether it is of high or low quality. So any inhibiting effect of the costs of distributing the information is now minimized.

Consideration of your personal situation and your preferences and values is important in making health care decisions. A person in midlife, with responsibility for children and their family, may be willing to endure treatments and procedures that have disagreeable side-effects and other costs in the quality of their life in order to maximize life-prolonging benefits. Older adults, however, usually express a preference for maintaining functional independence rather than having more intense medical management that could compromise their independence. **Spiritual** values such as dignity, religious beliefs, personal philosophy, and family relationships need to be considered as part of the equation when making medical choices.

An example that illustrates this is Emily, who is 34 years old and has a 5-year-old son. During her pregnancy, she developed a complication of pregnancy, called preeclampsia. She had high blood pressure and her kidney function was compromised. This complication resulted in her being hospitalized a month prior to her due date. She was treated with intravenous medications to lower her chances of having a stroke or of dying. She had a successful cesarean delivery. She still has high blood pressure that is controlled with medications, and her kidney function is mildly reduced. She is now 8 weeks into a second pregnancy. The chance of this pregnancy becoming complicated with preeclampsia again is high. She and her husband understand that this is a serious health threat, and must decide if they will continue or terminate the pregnancy. This is an example where spiritual and religious beliefs, as well as one's personal situation and family responsibilities, are factors that will influence the decision.

Time for reflection on the decision to be made and the different options being considered is necessary and almost always available. **Rarely are medical situations so urgent** that there is no time for "sleeping on" the options for several days or more. Our immediate reaction is just that, a reaction. Beware of pressure to make decisions quickly, such as when a surgeon says "the decision is up to you, but this condition is a time bomb," or this is a "window of opportunity for you to decide," with the suggestion that dire consequences will result if you do not decide in favor of an immediate intervention! When fear is a driving force in making a choice, it can cause you to react in an instinctive manner, with more chance of making an irrational decision. When you "sleep on" an issue which calls for a decision, you allow the brain to integrate the issues being considered, and as a result can have a deeper and clearer understanding of the situation.

Slowing down the process also allows more opportunity to mull your options over with people you trust and who care about you. Sometimes speaking with close friends or family can help you clarify your own preferences and values. This is best achieved when relying on people who are good at listening and asking questions, and who don't jump to their own conclusions or provide directions in an attempt to "fix" things for you.

The fourth factor is **having a clear understanding of the information available**. In the following chapters, we'll review examples of **recent research on the role of our emotions** in how we make medical decisions. We'll explore some common **misperceptions in how we view risk,** and how these misperceptions may color our understanding and influence our medical choices. Irrational thinking which is based on biases, beliefs, and feelings hinder the critical thinking necessary for making rational decisions.

Sometimes, belief can interfere with the clear understanding of medical information. For example, John and Barbara needed medical advice related to upcoming travel. They were going to Guatemala with their 4 and 6-year-old children for three months to work in a medical mission. Their children had not received the routine childhood immunizations because John and Barbara had feared their side-effects. They had read about some immunizations and chemicals in some vaccines being a possible cause of autism and had found websites and articles and television discussions that supported these beliefs. They were resistant to the recommendations that their children receive the standard childhood vaccines prior to their trip. The medical research and epidemiologic studies published in reputable medical journals have repeatedly shown that there is no link between vaccines and autism.

Unfortunately, a study that concluded that there was an association between autism and the vaccine for measles, mumps, and rubella, called the MMR vaccine, which received much publicity, was published in the highly regarded medical journal, **The Lancet** in 1998. This article was subsequently retracted by **The Lancet** due to evidence of research misconduct which invalidated the results, and sanctions to the author were applied in 2004. Yet the original study findings are still available in anti-immunization websites on the internet.

Immunizations have been one of the most effective public health interventions. In developing countries where immunization is less thoroughly practiced, there is a significantly higher incidence of these infectious diseases which can have severe consequences that include death. Standard childhood vaccines offer important protection against these illnesses and are especially important in parts of the world where these infectious diseases are more common. Yet John and Barbara were not open to considering the related medical information from recent scientific publications. Their concern about the side-effects of vaccines overwhelmed the information regarding their benefits. They did not realistically consider the risk of serious diseases that their travel would cause if their children were not vaccinated against them.

Personal beliefs, values, and life situation are factors to consider in making medical decisions. However, some beliefs can bias the information on which you are basing your decisions, and lead you to make choices that may fail to provide protection from risks that could be avoided. Be careful not to let your choice carry risks that have been shown to be avoidable, in an effort to avoid problems that do not have a scientific basis.

In the next chapter, we'll explore how people perceive risks and how this affects medical decision making.

Chapter 2

Perceptions of Risk

There are recognized patterns in how individuals regard risks. How we perceive risks we are facing can affect the decisions we make regarding our health care. The tendency is to simplify how we categorize risk. For example, we may see surgical options as always having more risk and personal costs than medications for the treatment of the same condition. This can cause us to make a decision without fully understanding all the potential ramifications. In this chapter, we'll consider some common misperceptions and simplifications of risk.

Risk is a term that is frequently used. **Risk** is defined as the possibility of an unwanted outcome. So one factor in how the concept of "risk" commonly used is the probability of an event or how likely is it to happen. However, the severity of the consequences of this unwanted outcome is important to consider as well. The probability of being infected by the HIV virus from one occasion of unprotected sex is low, but the infection will last a lifetime and may have serious consequences. Having a stroke, or heart attack, or dying, even if there is a low probability may still be a big risk because of the serious consequences. Being fatigued, or having a temporary ache, even if there is a high probability that it will occur, may be a small risk since the consequences are less severe. However, "risk" is often used interchangeably with "probability", especially when the unwanted outcome is described—for example, the risk of breast cancer refers to the probability of the occurrence of breast cancer. So, keep in mind that "risk" as we think of it in medical decision making, requires consideration of the likelihood of a problem occurring as well as the impact that problem could have on our life experience.

You need to understand that medical treatments are imperfect. A type of bias in the perception of risk is called **miscalibration.** In medical situations, this applies to **overconfidence about the extent and accuracy of medical treatments and knowledge**. This is understandable with the reports of so many scientific advances. Mapping of the human genome and the sophisticated work in precise molecular mechanisms and targeted treatments are examples of these amazing technical advances. Translating these advances into practical applications is a great challenge. Significant gaps still exist in medical knowledge.

It is common for this miscalibration to lead people to expect treatments to solve their problem or to lower the risk of a future event to zero. **There is a great appeal of zero risk**—no anxieties! But even well-accepted treatments only reduce risk. Treating hypertension or lowering cholesterol reduces the probability of a bad event such as a heart attack or stroke, but does not eliminate it. Treatment for a breast cancer only reduces the likelihood of a recurrence or the chance of it spreading. And treatments create their own problems and side effects that have to be considered.

So it is possible that the effort to lower a small risk associated with a health problem—to make it close to that appealing zero— exposes the person to an equal or greater risk from the treatment itself.

Consider the headline: "Aspirin cuts heart attack risks by 25%." You may ask: 25% of what? If the probability of having a heart attack in the next year is very small, then 25% of that number does not add up to very much. Let's consider the probability of an event such as a heart attack, which can be calculated using a valid formula developed to discern the probability of cardiovascular events like heart attacks or sudden death (see *Risk Calculators* in the supplements). In a group of one thousand 60-year-old men with normal blood pressure and average cholesterol, 8 or 9 of these men would be expected to have a heart attack in the next year. If each of these one thousand men took aspirin, only 6 or 7 of the thousand would have a heart attack. So to prevent one heart attack 500 men would need to take aspirin for a year. At the same time, it is calculated that one of these 500 men will have to be hospitalized due to bleeding (either intestinal or in the brain causing a stroke) as a side effect from taking the aspirin!

In contrast, consider a similar scenario in which the 1,000 men had elevated blood pressure and elevated cholesterol. Of this group, about 20 would be expected to have a heart attack in the next year. This number could be reduced to about 14 or 15 heart attacks if all the men took aspirin. So the difference in the effect of taking aspirin is greater (only 175 to 200 men would have to take aspirin for a year to prevent one heart attack), though in both scenarios the *risk reduction* is the same 25 percent.

Take another example: A woman was advised to take tamoxifen (a medication which blocks estrogen activity and is used to prevent the growth of breast cancer cells) by a breast cancer specialist at a major academic cancer center because she was at above average risk for breast cancer. She was told that taking tamoxifen would lower the probability of developing a breast cancer by about 40%. This is powerful advice from an authority at an important institution.

When we analyzed what the probability of her developing breast cancer was, it calculated that five out of one thousand women like her would develop cancer in a year. So she would lower her chance to three out of one thousand in a year by taking the medication (a 40% reduction). Again, 500 women like her would need to take tamoxifen for a year to prevent one of them from developing cancer. However, one of these 500 women taking tamoxifen would be expected to develop a serious complication from the medication, such as blood clots in her veins which might go into her lungs or cancer of the uterus. Perhaps you might consider breast cancer to be more serious and frightening, hence a bigger risk. It is important to know that the drug has frequent side effects that affect the quality of life, in addition to those serious complications, as well as financial costs that should be considered.

It was not an easy choice for her. The original recommendation came from an authoritative source with the best of intentions. Yet the thought of being on a medication and risking its side effects was a concern, too.

One tool you can use when facing a difficult choice is to try to change your perspective to the future and anticipate how you might feel by looking back from that perspective. This helps you to anticipate and avoid future feelings of **regret**. The "I should haves" are hard to live with, but can be anticipated by using this change of perspective.

After understanding the absolute numbers (500 women need to take the medicine to prevent one cancer) as opposed to the relative one—40% reduction—she found it useful to ask herself:
- How would I feel if I develop cancer even if I am taking tamoxifen?
- How would I feel if I develop one of the complications from the drug?
- How would I feel if I develop cancer if I do not take tamoxifen?

Another source of confusion in risk perception is **framing**: Is the glass half full or half empty?

How a situation is presented affects our reactions. Consider: You are walking down a street in a small city in Mexico where there are grates near some of the sidewalks give off a whiff of a foul smell as you walk past them. They are vents from the sewer and the smell can be offensive.

Now consider walking into a small cheese shop in Paris. That very similar smell of fermentation in this shop may now be quite enticing. The smell may be the same, but the frame has changed.

The interpretation of medical data is greatly affected by the formulation of the presentation, or of the frame used to present it. A middle-aged man is diagnosed with early lung cancer and surgery is recommended. The statistics for 100 men undergoing this surgery can be presented to this patient as:

- 90 will live through the surgery and first postoperative month and 34 will be alive at the end of 5 years.

Alternatively:
- 10 will die within the first month and 66 will be dead after 5 years.

The facts are not different, but how they are presented can make a world of difference. One formulation is more frightening than the other: "10 dying in the first month" is more impressive since the difference from 0 to 10 dying seems proportionately greater than the difference of 90 out of 100 surviving. Framing effects are difficult to eliminate because information is always presented in a frame. Patients and physicians can be swayed by the choice of one formulation or another.

There are three useful strategies to counteract this influence. You may need to devise the presentation of these strategies yourself if your doctor does not present the information in different frames for you.
- Consider the data from different perspectives or frames. How many people of the total suffer complications from an intervention vs. how many people do well? If the different perspectives do not alter how you react to the information, you can be more comfortable with the decision. If the reactions diverge, then you should continue exploring the information.
- Use a visual aid. Some people are better at gaining comprehension visually so a chart with stick figures of different colors that represent different outcomes, for example, can prove enlightening (See Figure 1).
- Discuss the situation with someone who has a different perspective or opinion and see if you can be swayed. Ask them to be a "devil's advocate" for you, to reframe the situation.

Figure 1

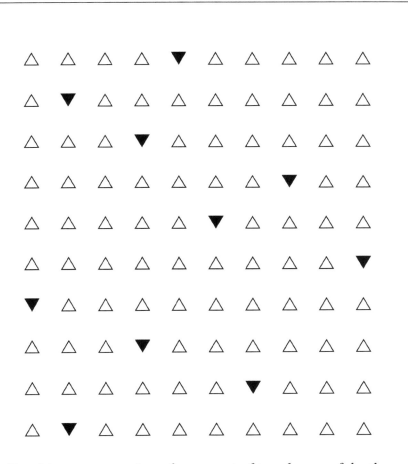

Graphic representation of a one out of ten chance of death (black Figures)

Another way we tend to **simplify the perception of risk is a categorical judgment that something is good or bad, safe or dangerous**. Making such "either-or" judgments simplifies things. But this rarely leads to an informed, carefully considered conclusion.

There are very few absolutely good or absolutely bad things. *In actuality, the dose or amount of exposure is the determining factor in the safety or risk of anything.*

Is a small bowl of ice-cream harmful? Many people would answer yes, yet a quart of yogurt or cottage cheese which has many more calories and much more fat is considered healthy. Medications like antibiotics, in too low a dose, may cause side effects and bacterial resistance without resolving the infection being treated, yet in a dose too high, there may be harmful side effects. The right dose may speed healing while minimizing these side effects.

People commonly believe that we cannot ingest too many vitamins since they are necessary and beneficial and safe. But the dose of any particular type of vitamin will determine benefit or harm. There is solid evidence too much vitamin A, vitamin D, vitamin C, folic acid, niacin, pyridoxine, or iron, can cause harm. This has been demonstrated through many long-term studies using these supplements in sick and well persons.

Most people are familiar with the dangers of alcohol. Yet, we now know that moderate alcohol ingestion by people over 50 is associated with a lowered mortality. The effect of alcohol on mortality is, in reality, a J-shaped curve, with the lowest mortality associated with having 1-½ drinks per day (at the bottom of the J), those who drink less have a higher mortality (go up the small arm of the J to the left) and those who drink more go up the big arm of the J towards rising mortality to the right. (See the figure 2 below as an example of a J-shaped curve which is evident in various health related measures including measures of obesity.) While overuse of alcohol is the most dangerous pattern, teetotalers do not get the health benefits that result with moderate alcohol consumption.

So, specific doses or levels of exposure to medications, nutrients, and other substances or situations can pose a risk at times and be beneficial at other times. Generally, *moderation* is a concept and approach worth embracing and is a safer bet than approaching things in absolute terms, categorizing them as all good or all bad.

Figure 2

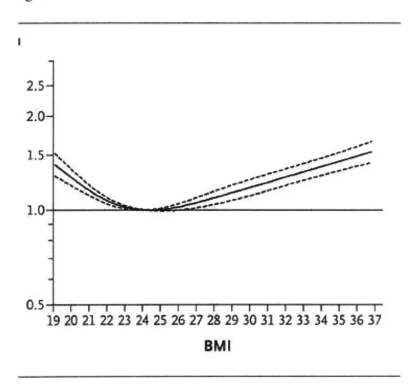

An example of a J-Shaped Curve, sometimes called a "U-Shaped Curve," for the relative risk of death as BMI (a measure of obesity) varies. The relative risk of death is on the vertical axis.

Chapter 3

Emotions and Bias

We have been focusing on how having an understanding of the factors that influence the decisions you make can improve your ability to make wise decisions in health care. This helps you choose options for your medical condition that are best suited to your values and preferences. In this chapter, we'll examine how common feelings can impair our ability to make wise choices. These feelings can bias or prejudice our choices by interfering with our ability to remain clear-headed in assessing the options available. This is particularly true when we are uncertain what the impact might be on our health and well-being as a result of choosing one or other of the different options available to us.

A common bias when looking at information is called **confirmation bias**.

We have beliefs, ideas, and opinions, and our brain tries to find evidence to substantiate them. So we select information that supports our pre-conceived notions or perceptions and tend to avoid or ignore information which opposes them.

Politicians as a group often provide examples of the effects of this bias, and as a result, make decisions that are not critically considered and may turn out to be harmful. When leaders surround themselves with people who will only agree with them, and avoid presenting differing views, it can lead to dangerous decisions. This is one manifestation of confirmation bias. Former President George W. Bush's decision to invade Iraq was a clear example of this bias. How many reasons did we hear to support the opinion that it was the right decision? And whenever one of the reasons was disproved, another reason was found to "confirm" the original argument.

This bias, which we all tend toward, often leads to relying on skewed information in our decision making. Patients may go from one consultant to another until they get the opinion or the prescription they believe is best, confirming their opinions. Physicians do this, too. They may have an opinion about a diagnosis or treatment early in the course of their decision making and seek those tests and data that support their initial conclusion and tend to confirm it. To reach the best decision, attention must be given to opposing views and information, as well as to information that is supportive.

Another form of confirmation bias is seen in the lack of critical appraisal of the information that supports one's view. Philip was convinced that vitamin C helped him avoid infections with respiratory viruses that cause colds. He cited an article which showed that mice which were given large doses of vitamin C were more resistant to viral infections than ones not provided this supplement. This small study was the basis of his decision to use vitamin C. He ignored the fact that he is not a mouse, and that many other studies in humans have not shown such protection. Critical thinking requires open-minded consideration of a variety of views and information, regardless of what position the information may support.

Predicting future feelings is difficult. When we have a choice to make, we try to imagine what it will feel like to experience the different possible outcomes. We have experience of the present and the past but can only imagine the future. The way we feel right now is the way we think we will feel in the future. People fail to anticipate how their preferences and feelings may change over time.

Humans are very adaptable. In a study by Brinkman and Coates (cited in the *References*) that illustrates this adaptability, individuals rated their quality of life one year after winning a lottery. Another group rated their quality of life one year after an accident which had left them paraplegic. The ratings provided by these two groups, a year after what nearly everyone would consider being wildly different luck in life, were basically the same. The adaptation to what looked like great news and the adaptation to disastrous news brought people back to their common, original way of feeling about their lives. These two groups indicated they would not have predicted prior to the event that they would feel as they did, one year later.

Consider the following situation: A man is diagnosed with rectal cancer and must decide whether to undergo surgery which will result in a colostomy. This means that part of his colon will be removed and his remaining bowel would empty into a bag attached to his abdomen. He had a strong aversive reaction to this suggestion initially. It is important for him to consider not only how he will react immediately after the surgery, but how he will adapt, and how his current concerns will fade over time. So he needs to understand both how his life will change with a colostomy, and how his attitude to it will subsequently change. It can be very helpful in a situation like this to talk to someone who has undergone that very same operation, and try to anticipate his own future feelings after hearing about their experience around this surgery, and how they felt about the results over time. Surveys show that for most patients, one year after a colostomy their ratings of their quality of life return to the pre-operative baseline. Yet most people would not predict this result.

Another common shortcut used in making decisions is called the **availability bias**. This bias becomes evident when we react to information that is currently *available* in our minds and thoughts. What makes it available?

Consider Miriam's case. She has a damaged right knee from a congenital misalignment which has eroded all of her cartilage. She has a lot of pain whenever she walks, and as a result is less active. She has gained weight and also has strained her relationship with her spouse since she cannot do much housework, nor go on walks which have been an important part of their shared lives. Her pain, in addition, makes her irritable.

She has consulted with two orthopedic surgeons who feel that a total knee replacement offers the only way to be able to walk pain-free.

She is naturally anxious about this procedure, but after reviewing her options, discussing it with her spouse and others, she decides it is reasonable to proceed.

In mentioning this upcoming surgery to her neighbor across the street, he tells her he had that procedure at the same hospital where she is scheduled to have her surgery, and that he feels it was a big mistake for him. He had a lot of pain right after the surgery. Then his knee replacement became loose so they had to revise the knee with another procedure. It was still painful and still not fully stable so he underwent two additional procedures to correct this. He has never been able to walk comfortably since his surgery. "I'd never go through that again."

His vivid description scares Miriam into canceling her surgery. It is a vivid and **available** anecdote and tends to **confirm** her prior anxieties. Instead of seeking additional information about the broad experience with this procedure, she chose to forego the operation and has been going to an alternative medicine practitioner who is injecting a homeopathic medicine into the tissue around the knee. Miriam says that maybe it feels a little better.

As we know, no medical procedure or treatment is risk-free. But the rates of possible complications of knee replacements that her orthopedists quoted are based on 300,000-500,000 such surgeries each year, and they are infrequent. The complication that her neighbor suffered would not affect the overall numbers, but this vivid story altered Miriam's view of her risks and caused her to make a decision not based on the actual probability of her experiencing any problems.

Vivid memories of our own experiences or of people close to us, such as family members, are *available*. Vivid anecdotes of others' experiences with procedures or problems similar to the one we are facing are *available*. Also, those topics that have received notoriety through prominent news coverage come to our minds easily. We tend to **markedly overestimate** the probability of experiencing a problem we could be at risk for if that problem is *available* in our mind. A group of 50 to 52-year-old women were asked to estimate their risk of having breast cancer over the next 15 years. This is a subject that is frequently in the news, either because of famous people who are reported to suffer from it, or because there are newsworthy medical stories about this common serious illness. It may also be *available* because we may know people who have had such a diagnosis. There is a lot of interest in this condition. These women estimated their risk at an average of 50%. Yet the reality is dramatically different. The actual risk is closer to 5%.

Attribution bias is another shortcut that can limit our focus when considering causes of symptoms or problems. This happens when a person with a previously diagnosed condition has a new discomfort that they *attribute* to the previously diagnosed condition. For example, a person with a history of irritable bowel syndrome, a condition that causes recurrent discomfort in the abdomen and changes in bowel function develops abdominal pain. They may consider it just part of their syndrome. Yet abdominal pain may be caused by an entirely different condition. A headache may be attributed to an old pattern of tension-type headaches, yet there could be another cause. This is a way of simplifying the considerations, yet if the new symptoms are a little different, more prolonged, or concerning, we must allow other possibilities to be considered.

Daniel was diagnosed with an aggressive lymphoma and was given six cycles of chemotherapy. The treatment successfully induced a remission of his cancer. He spent a year gradually regaining his strength and he felt he had regained 80% of the quality of life he had prior to the diagnosis and treatment. Three years after the initial diagnosis, during a routine surveillance done after such a cancer, a new growth was noted. A small biopsy was done which was positive for lymphatic cancer.

The oncologist (cancer specialist) who provided the initial treatment program attributed this new growth to be a recurrence of the initial cancer. A new and very aggressive treatment protocol was suggested which would include a bone marrow transplant. Daniel went for a second opinion to look for alternative treatments at another health care facility specializing in lymphatic cancers. They suggested a second biopsy of the abnormal node to ascertain if this was the original cancer that had recurred. A more extensive biopsy was carefully examined, and this revealed that this was a new and different cancer. This one was less aggressive and would require treatment that had many less adverse consequences than the very aggressive approach recommended by his first oncologist.

Occam's razor is the principle that states that the simplest explanation is usually the correct one. That means one diagnosis is more likely to be the cause of multiple symptoms than several different problems occurring at one time. But this is not always the case, of course. The other possibility is sometimes referred to as **Hickam's Dictum.** John Hickam was the chairman of Indiana University's Internal Medicine Department in the 1950s and he stated: "Patients can have as many diseases as they damn well please" at one time—in opposition to the parsimony of Occam's Razor. He reasoned that several common diseases are more likely to be present at the same time than one less common ailment in a single patient causing a variety of symptoms. The bottom line: do not jump to conclusions before carefully examining the data.

Another tendency that can bias decisions is the **preference for the status quo**. People are reluctant to relinquish their current routines. Change can make us anxious.

George has been taking vitamin E for the last 15 years, following his doctor's advice years ago when they were discussing ways to lower his risk of having a heart attack. Vitamin E is an anti-oxidant vitamin which has been a popular supplement. Its use is suggested because oxidation is important in the aging process, and because oxidation is felt to be involved in cancer promotion, arteriosclerosis, and the decline of cognitive and mental abilities. New evidence, however, not only suggests that vitamin E is ineffective in preventing these problems, but may actually increase the chance of developing heart failure and dying. When his current doctor suggested he stop taking the supplement, George was reluctant. Things had gone well, and it was part of his daily routine. He felt that it was protecting him. He is not alone in this reluctance since many scientists and doctors have a similar reaction. They attempt to find fault with new evidence in order to justify an established behavior such as continuing to take a supplement containing Vitamin E. This reluctance to change our behavior (which includes reluctance to stop taking medicines that we feel have been protecting us) is common when new information shows that some treatments may be ineffective, wasteful, or harmful.

This reaction is very common with medicines used to treat problems that may be present for a limited time, such as hormonal conditions, gastrointestinal problems like constipation and heartburn, as well as pain. Sometimes a problem we have had is fully resolved—like an ulcer—yet we fear it may recur if we stop taking the pill that helped us recover. So we don't stop, even though there is no ongoing medical need for the treatment, and continuing an unnecessary medication exposes us to possible harmful side-effects.

It can be frightening to stop taking medicines. Frequently, doctors add new ones but rarely discontinue the old. They also have difficulties in stopping old medications, even when the benefits are not clear. The phenomenon of taking increasing numbers of medicines over time is common. The older we get, the more pills we take. Some of this is due to having more medical conditions, but it can also be due to the **preference for the status quo**. Taking many different medications can be confusing, and increases the chances of drug interactions and side effects. It is also more expensive.

Benjamin visited his doctor because he was feeling fatigued, "old" for his age, and unwell. As part of the consultation, he was asked what medicines and other pills he was taking. Besides several prescriptions for a heart rhythm problem and for prostate cancer, he was taking 38 different supplements by mouth. In addition, he was getting intravenous infusions of supplements on a weekly basis. He would add a new supplement when different people he talked to told him it was the best way to help him live longer and better. But he never discontinued taking any of the earlier ones because he feared he would lose whatever benefit they may be giving. As a result, a number of the supplements were having opposing effects, and others were interfering with his prescribed medications. He was even having allergic reactions to some of these supplements. All of this while spending several hundred dollars a month on these treatments.

Benjamin was able to discontinue a number of them after discussing how these pills were worked against each other and against his prescriptions and after considering new evidence of potential harm associated with particular supplements. But, it was worrisome for him to do this, and he could only do it gradually and with persistent encouragement to do so. After several months, he was taking one fourth of the original number and had stopped the intravenous infusions. He said he felt better! However, his wife reports that the number of supplements he is taking is gradually increasing again.

Some tendencies, though not rational, are hard to change. It can be that this difficulty is precisely because they aren't rational. Think about your own health and self-care behaviors and beliefs. Which of them are rational, which aren't? Which are based on sound evidence of added benefits, which aren't? Which, if any, do you hold on to for fear of letting go?

One strategy to decrease the tendency to "prefer the status quo" is to suggest and discuss the situation from a different reference point. For example, George might be asked to imagine that this was his first visit to the doctor for a consultation. His question is: what treatments and approaches should he start with to lower his chance of having a heart attack? His doctor could point out that he certainly would not suggest vitamin E to be part of his risk lowering strategy if he was a new patient asking this question. The goal with this approach would be to change the reference point in his thought process. Rather starting with the *status quo* (which for him includes the use of vitamin E, which he considers "normal"), he'd be asked to think of the problem as if he were starting from scratch, which is a very different vantage point. Considering the issue from another perspective, or reference point can provide new insight on a given health problem or health behavior.

Here is a non-medical example to illustrate how changing the reference point can provide a new perspective. Flying from Detroit to Los Angeles takes about 41/2 hours. Another 2½ hours is needed to drive to the airport, go through security and wait to take off. Then there is still the time required at the rental-car desk after arriving in Los Angeles and the drive from the airport to the final destination, another hour or more—for a total of about 8-9 hours. One knows what to expect in this long process, yet unexpected minor delays can cause great annoyance. How does it feel when you go to retrieve your suitcase at the baggage claim on such a trip, to encounter a delay of 15 minutes before the bags are delivered? What if you notice that bags from flights that arrived after yours are already on the luggage carousel? Might that get under your skin and cause frustration and anxiety? That is a common reaction. Yet, if you change your reference point from the delay in your bag arrival time to the overall travel time—8-9 hours, it might help you realize that the bag delay had only a minimal impact, and really isn't that important. Sometimes perspective, or the way you view experiences or decisions, can make all the difference in how we feel.

Changing behaviors, like diet and exercise routines, is sometimes difficult because of the **preference for the *status quo***. Runners are often unwilling to stop their routines even after developing injuries from "overuse" due to their running. They fear the loss of fitness, the ability to maintain their weight, and other benefits. It may be helpful to describe how different exercises, or equally healthy but more moderate routines, may give them the same net health benefits. Seeing change this way may ease their anxiety about making a modification that would be beneficial (a different reference point).

Irrational Reactions

Emotions when facing a choice are sometimes intense. In such cases, people may realize that the **reaction is irrational**, yet remain unable to reconcile their priorities. Consider the reaction of **disgust**.

You may be interested to know that there are academics that specialize in the study of disgust! They will design experiments intended to elicit disgust. For example, they will have a pitcher of punch and stir it with a plastic spoon before offering it to the subjects. People do not seem to have any problem drinking this punch. No disgust! But when the pitcher is stirred with a new plastic fly swatter just removed from its wrapper, many people would not drink the punch. The association of a fly swatter, even a new and clean one, with the drink, elicited disgust. Disgust can affect decisions even in situations where we recognize that it is an irrational reaction. There are many situations in medicine which elicit disgust in people, and hence can influence their decisions. Parts of our bodies and products or secretions from these can elicit disgust and may cause us to avoid thinking or considering health issues that revolve around these.

A medical example of this irrational reaction can be seen in cancer screening. In the US 75% of men over 50 years old have had a PSA (prostate-specific antigen) test to detect possible prostate cancer. Having this simple blood test done has not been shown to lead to living longer or to lowering the chance of dying from prostate cancer. Yet fewer than 50% of adults over 50 have had tests to detect colon cancer, even though it has been convincingly shown that having such a test results in a lower chance of having colon cancer and of dying from colon cancer. These colon cancer screening tests involve either testing feces for hidden blood or having a procedure with a long scope inserted into the anus to examine the colon and rectum. The aversive reaction to the tests is not rational. It goes against the evidence of benefits from the screening procedures. Yet it can be very strong. Far too few men and women have colon cancer screening, in large part because of their irrational discomfort with the tests, which in part stems from a feeling of disgust.

How we manage **worry** can influence health behaviors and decisions. Worry can motivate us to be careful and to follow healthy lifestyles and to comply with our treatment plans. Excessive worry can paralyze some people with fear, though. A common method of worry management is the denial of problems or symptoms, avoiding health care altogether. Some people will deny that smoking and other recognized unhealthy behaviors pose risks to them in order not to worry. Some women deliberately avoid seeking medical attention after noticing a lump in the breast. Excessive worry about what may be found leads them to deny that it needs to be evaluated.

I was part of a medical group traveling to China which included a psychiatrist. He jogged every morning for 20 minutes, even though he was an object of curiosity for the Chinese. He also smoked 8-10 cigarettes each day. I asked him how can it be that a disciplined jogger like him could smoke. "Why do you think I jog?" he answered. "To cancel the effects of smoking!" Even an expert in irrational behaviors and thinking was not immune to them!

Here's a description of a funny medical cartoon, which illustrates the effects of anxieties and irrational concerns on our understanding of medical information: A patient is sitting on an exam table listening to the doctor's explanation. The doctor is standing next to him with his chart and had just given him the reasoning for the diagnosis for his concerns. The patient replies: "It makes a lot of sense, doctor, that really my problem is that I am a hypochondriac. But tell me; couldn't that condition be caused by a brain tumor?"

Section 2

The Process

Relationships involve more than a single individual, of course. Each person involved in a relationship has a role to play. But these roles may be unbalanced, with one person having more power and influence or much more responsibility than the other. Relationships can impact medical decision making as well.

Clearly, between a child and parent, decision making is not fully shared, since there is a hierarchy in the family, and children have neither the legal authority nor, in most instances, the maturity to make medical decisions. There may be other power imbalances in the family, such as between a husband and a wife, which can affect medical decision making. With our health care providers, traditionally, our relationships have been unbalanced. This can lead to the patient giving up opportunities to be fully heard, to play an important part in making decisions, and to share responsibility for the consequences.

This section presents information on the structure of health care which can lead to some imbalance in the relationship between doctor and patient. Ideas and tools on being a full participant when interacting with your doctor are presented. Your doctors can benefit from your consideration and understanding of their roles in this relationship. You can help them provide the best health care for you and your family. You will need to advocate for your interests and be comfortable in asking questions, even if they seem hard or pointed. By having an understanding of each person's role in this process, and compassion for all participants, you can be empowered to become a thoughtful advocate for yourself and your family.

Consumerism as a social and economic order encourages the acquisition of goods and services and is a potent force in the functioning of our economy. We are aware that excess consumption can also lead to social and environmental harm. When consumerism impacts medical care, it can be a source of diminishing the quality of care. The way medicine is practiced and marketed in the United States encourages the utilization of more care which is not necessarily better care. Being able to assertively and carefully question your health care provider will decrease the chance that you will receive unnecessary diagnostic tests, procedures or prescriptions. I discuss this in a chapter of this section.

Chapter 4
Going to the Doctor

In this chapter, we'll explore the process of visiting a doctor. How do you feel when you have decided to go to the doctor? Are you prepared to describe your concerns to the doctor? How does that process of the visit unfold and how does it affect the way you make decisions? Do you truly understand the decisions and plans you and your doctor have made? Are you comfortable with these choices and do they seem logical? What common patterns do visits to doctors take?

Preparing for the visit enhances your ability to speak clearly and to be heard. In addition, there are tools to make your visits more effective and complete, as well as ideas on how to remember the discussion you had during the visit. This includes clearly remembering the plans and goals that were offered and made, as well as the reasoning behind them. We will also consider here what additional support would make it more likely that your visit will fully satisfy your needs.

No one goes to the doctor for fun. Yet, a visit to a doctor is often a necessary first step when making personal medical decisions. Going to the doctor is often associated with discomforts, with a sense of anxiety and fear, and with feelings of being dependent and powerless. The way modern health care is structured does not make it easy for you to participate in making health care choices. The medical establishment is centered more on the needs of the health care providers and their institutions with the intention of maximizing the efficiency of the operation of their clinics, rather than meeting the needs of patients. This can create an environment in which full and active participation by the patient and their loved ones with their medical providers is more difficult.

Barriers to Covering all Your Concerns During a Visit

Patients express great dissatisfaction at long waiting times and short consultations. Studies show that the length of time spent with the doctor has remained about the same in the U.S. over the past two decades, averaging from 14 to 22 minutes. The length depends, in part, on the nature of the concerns (more complex problems require more time), the gender of the clinician (women clinicians, on average, spend two minutes in each visit more than men), the payment scheme (pre-paid visits are shorter than fee-for-service visits), and other factors. However, what has changed in recent years is the perception by both clinicians and patients that visits are more rushed, leaving less than adequate time for properly exploring all the problems in each visit. This is, in part, due to the increased paperwork and bureaucracy involved in the practice of medicine today. There are more government and insurance requirements. For example, approvals are sometimes required for medications or tests or other procedures. Now in addition to office visits, there are emails and telephone calls requiring a response. Demands for the doctors to be more productive (to see more patients) have become increasingly transparent. So even if the length of the visit has remained the same, the tension caused by not having enough time has increased for patients and for doctors. Doctors today express increased frustration over the demands of their practice.

Visits to a doctor have limited time allotments to cover all your concerns and to complete the required documentation. So the opportunity to state all you want to discuss during the visit is limited. One study which observed the practices of experienced family physicians revealed that *patients completely stated their concerns in only 28% of visits*. The two main reasons that people did not state all the issues they wanted to discuss during the visit were:

1) They were not initially asked why they had come to see the doctor and so did not get an opportunity to list their concerns, or

2) Patients were *redirected* during the initial explanation of the purpose of their visit by the doctor.

This "redirection" happens when the physician interrupts a patient before they have completed their reasons for coming to see the doctor. While you are beginning to state what brought you to this visit, something in that description catches the physician's attention and he *redirects* all the attention to this. The visit then stays on this concern or simply on the items you had mentioned before the doctor first interrupted you. In this study, *the mean time the patients had to express their concern as the visit began before the physician redirected the focus was only 23.1 seconds*! Once the discussion became focused on a specific concern, patients were able to return to other issues and complete their agendas in only 8% of visits!

Brian went to see his doctor to follow up on his back pain and high blood pressure. When the doctor asked him how he was feeling, he started by mentioning that he had had several episodes of pain in his abdomen recently. Brian had wanted to discuss his back pain and blood pressure medications as well. He even wondered if they might be related to the abdominal pain. But the doctor focused on this initial statement and began to ask him about the timing and character of the pain. Was it related to foods or bowel movements? After spending time describing his abdominal pain, Brian lost his initial train of thought and realized well after leaving the office that while he had expected to discuss his back pain and blood pressure, they never got around to his main issues. The doctor covered what he felt to be of greater importance, requested Brian return in 6 months, and prepared to see his next patient.

Difficulties Remembering and Understanding the Advice

The anxieties and tension that affect most people when seeing a doctor may make it difficult to pay full attention to the physician's information and instructions. It is generally accepted that 50% or less of instructions received in a visit with a health care provider will be recalled immediately following the visit, and the percentage remembered decreases further a short time after the visit. Studies reveal that, depending on the type of advice, there is a recall of 20%-70% of these instructions after two or three days. Greater numbers of instructions mean less is remembered, and more complex instructions are more difficult to remember.

Mary was told she had an elevated cholesterol level. Proceeding according to well-accepted guidelines she was advised by her doctor to take medications to lower the cholesterol in addition to starting a diet low in saturated and trans fats. She was prescribed a "statin" medication to lower the cholesterol and received dietary advice from a nutritionist. She was given a pamphlet with dietary information on lowering cholesterol. When she returned 6 weeks later for a check up, she had stopped taking her medications and was barely adhering to her diet. She said that she had understood that the statins would take care of the cholesterol problem, and had taken the entire prescription which was written for one month (her insurance plan required the medication to be dispensed this way, with the need to have the prescription refilled each month in order to continue taking the medication). She believed she had followed all the instructions. What she did not understand was that the cholesterol elevation was a chronic condition requiring ongoing medication and diet to maintain control. It cannot be cured by taking one course of medicines. She had never considered refilling her prescription, even though it had called for monthly renewals. She was not alone in her relaxed approach to the nutritionist's advice, as less than 10% of patients follow dietary recommendations closely for more than a few months!

Health care providers are taught that when patients have problems controlling their diabetes, elevated blood pressure, or other chronic conditions, the most likely explanation is their failure to adhere to the medical program. We are now learning that not fully understanding at the outset the language the doctor uses to explain the problem and the treatment, forgetting instructions, not fully understanding the nature of the condition, and complex treatment programs which may be hard to follow are some of the factors that make adhering to a management plan more difficult. It is not just that patients are being difficult!

Instructions are often hard to understand. The ability to read and understand health care information varies widely. Studies of patients' understanding of instructions have shown that people who understood explanations and instructions least, had poorer physical and psychological health, incurred greater health care costs, and had poorer control of chronic conditions like diabetes and hypertension. Simple instructions such as how frequently to take medications and whether to take them on an empty stomach or not were understood by only 19% of English-speaking patients seen at one U.S. public hospital. In addition, most of the patients who were unclear about the instructions did not ask for more explanation. They often said they felt shame in admitting that they did not understand.

Preparing Ourselves for a Visit to the Doctor

How can we improve the process and create the conditions that make going to the doctor more fruitful? Prepare for your visit by thinking through your goals for the visit ahead of time, and list them in writing several days before seeing the doctor. This way you can amend and add to the list as a way of preparing. In thinking of each item, you might look for new ideas and information about some of them, and so prepare yourself to discuss them. Discussing your list with a friend or family member in advance, particularly if your health problems and questions are complex, can also be a big help in clarifying what you need to learn and what you want to accomplish. If you bring the written list of concerns and information with you to your visit, it is less likely that you will forget or be diverted (or redirected) from raising your concerns and having these addressed.

It is also a good opportunity before the visit to review your priorities. Then, if your doctor suggests diagnostic tests, such as a stress test, sleep study, a cancer screen, or other procedures (that have been used unnecessarily in some sectors of the population such as the elderly), you can be prepared to ask how the results of the tests will be used to manage your care. Do they seem to fit with what you see as your goals or priorities? You can ask, "Do you feel this test or procedure or treatment will truly be helpful for me?" and "what are the chances the tests may give false positive results leading to a more intrusive testing cascade going forward?"

You should also be prepared to **tell your health care provider you will need time to consider their suggestions.** Processing the recommendations at home removes the distractions we face in the doctor's office. Slowing the process allows you to carefully consider your reactions.

Having someone accompany you is another way of lessening the intensity of feelings around the medical visit. Just the **support** provided by having a companion can be significant. In addition, having two sets of ears and two brains at work on your behalf can increase the chances of understanding and remembering what is said. It is surprising how frequently two people listening to the same material hear different information and instructions, and remember different parts more clearly. When the issues are complex or overwhelming, going to a visit with a companion or advocate offers great advantages. This is particularly the case when the visit is due to an unexpected or urgent concern, or when you are in pain or are in discomfort.

Joe had always been a vigorous and healthy man. Even in his mid 60's, he was still jogging four miles every morning. Early one dark morning when he was jogging, he twisted his ankle on the curb edge and fell. The severe pain told him it was serious. At the emergency room, a fracture was found on the x-ray and he was scheduled to see an orthopedic surgeon the next day. His brother accompanied him to that visit to help with driving and ambulation. When the orthopedist evaluated him and told Joe he needed surgery to stabilize the ankle, he was stunned and frightened. All he could focus on was how suddenly he had gone from being able and independent to being incapacitated. He even needed an operation, which was frightening. His feelings about this caused him to be unable to focus on the explanations and instructions to prepare for his procedure the next day. Fortunately, his brother was able to pay attention to the explanation, and ask questions about the procedure and how to prepare for the operation, what the risks were, how long he would need to be off his leg, what was the typical time for healing, and what the follow-up plans would be. That evening, Joe's brother reminded him of simple and practical measures he needed to follow prior to the surgery, such as why not to eat anything after midnight to be ready for the anesthesia.

This is an example of how a companion can be helpful in getting the medical care you need, and in understanding the explanations and plans. Your feelings when you are in pain or afraid, or even simply surprised by the news, can make it difficult to pay full attention to the doctor. It is easy, in these cases, to forget simple instructions, and it can make it very difficult to ask for the clarifications you may need to follow the treatment plans. A companion can provide you the time and space you need to settle down and gain some perspective on the situation. Joe had his surgery, and he recovered as the doctor had predicted.

Preparing the Doctor for Your Visit

Preparing the medical practitioner for your agenda is another way of increasing the benefits of a visit. Doctors always do this when referring a patient to a colleague, providing information to the consultant about the patient's condition and the questions being raised in advance of the visit. Harold had an appointment to see his primary care provider for a follow-up of his heart condition. He tried to be aware of medical advances and had read of new treatments being considered for patients with similar heart problems, and wondered if he might benefit from these new approaches. He sent his doctor an email saying that he would be seeing her in a few weeks and mentioning that he would value her opinion on these novel approaches. During his visit, the doctor described the studies on which Harold's information was based that led to new treatments for people with his condition, and how these might be beneficial for him. When Harold thanked her for her diligence and the work she had done in preparing for his visit, she said: "My pleasure. It gave me a chance to bone up on these new developments. It provided me with a nice change of routine, and it was quite stimulating."

Presenting the list of your concerns in advance enables your doctor to think about the issues, perhaps to do some research on them, and consult with other colleagues. Rather than being surprised by the questions, the medical practitioner has the opportunity to have the comfort and satisfaction of being a well-informed expert and guide. It is also more likely that redirection will not take place, therefore allowing your full agenda to be considered.

Help in Understanding and Remembering

Having a clear understanding of the plans for diagnostic testing and treatment is important for patients. It increases the likelihood that the patient will follow the recommendations. Writing the information down as it is given can reduce the chance of not remembering it later. Once you have taken notes, you are more able to pay full attention to what is being said, since you do not have to worry about remembering every detail. The note taker can be either you or someone who accompanies you. You may also ask the doctor if you could tape record his recommendations and plans, as a memory aid, if that is more comfortable for you.

What comes after the visit? How and when can you expect results? How will you be informed? If tests or procedures have been done, waiting to learn of the results can cause great anxiety and discomfort. Having clear mechanisms for obtaining results and having follow-up plans can minimize this source of stress. Asking the health care provider how you can best advise him of any changes that appear important is helpful. Ask specific questions, like: "Can I email you information? Is a telephone call a better way of staying in touch? How long does it usually take to receive a reply or a return call? What changes in my condition do you feel would be important to let you know of right away?" Preparing for the medical visit, having help in remembering and understanding the explanation, being accompanied and supported, and keeping notes are useful tools that make it more likely you will be able to adhere to the program recommended and get the most benefit out of the health care you receive.

It may feel uncomfortable to be assertive. You may feel you are imposing yourself in what feels like a "pushy" manner. It may feel like you are not being a "good" patient. Polite assertiveness, however, provides an opportunity to be clear about what your concerns and preferences are as a patient. It also provides an opportunity for doctors to prepare and to clarify what you can expect from them and their staff. If you know what the preferred process is for continuing your health care, you are more likely not to cause surprises and discomforts for yourself, or your health care providers. Of course, wisdom and courtesy in framing your concerns, questions, and preferences always enhances the relationships between patients and doctors. Expressions of thanks and courtesy go a long way to making it enjoyable and engaging for both you and your doctor.

Chapter 5

More Care is not Necessarily Better Care

Your goal is to receive the highest quality medical care available. It is clear that the quality of health care has been, and continues to be lowered by misuse of medical technology and medications. Using radiation to treat acne, as was done decades ago is an example of the misuse of technology that caused harm. Side effects, including cases of thyroid cancer, caused great suffering. These side effects of radiation were not fully recognized at the time. Later it became clear that this is a form of misuse of medical technology. Underuse of health care resources also lowers the quality of health care. It is logical that not having a needed diagnostic test, or not receiving appropriate medication are examples of poor quality health care. You may not realize, though, that the overuse of health care resources can also result in poor quality of care as well. You may be surprised to know that this is a common occurrence in the United States. Let's look at some of the reasons that overuse lowers the quality of care, as well as why more services than necessary are frequently utilized.

Pamela told her doctor during her annual physical examination that since she underwent a screening colonoscopy the previous year (the results were normal) she had been experiencing episodes of pain and discomfort in her abdomen. The discomfort was difficult to describe. Sometimes it felt like a stitch in her right side, sometimes she felt constipated and gassy. It did not interfere with her sleeping, nor had she lost weight. Her doctor examined her, ordered blood tests and urine tests, all of which were normal. Then he suggested that she have an ultrasound of her abdomen; it might reveal the cause of her discomfort. The ultrasound revealed two stones in her gall bladder. Perhaps that was the cause of her discomforts, her doctor thought and referred her to a surgeon for a consultation.

The surgeon thought it possible that the gallstones were causing her abdominal symptoms. He recommended a CT (computerized tomography) scan of the abdomen to "rule out" other problems and to confirm the ultrasound findings. Her CT scan confirmed her gallstones and also revealed a small mass or growth on her right adrenal gland. He advised her to consult an endocrinologist, since the adrenal mass could be a tumor that produced abnormal amounts of hormones. The endocrinologist ordered biochemical analysis of the adrenal hormones, which were normal. The endocrinologist advised that, although the mass was currently quite small and unlikely to be dangerous or cause symptoms presently, it be monitored periodically to see if it grew.

She returned to see the surgeon, who suggested removing her gall bladder since the stones in the gall bladder were an abnormality that might be causing her symptoms. He reasoned that even if the current discomfort was not due to the gallstones, she might develop problems from them in the future.

By checking some sites on the internet and by looking at some medical texts, Pamela found statistics that revealed that 20% of women over 40 (she is 56 years old) have gallstones, yet only 1% ever develops typical gall bladder attacks. Removing the gall bladder for symptoms that are not specific for gall bladder attacks usually, does not relieve the symptoms. Gall bladder surgery, like any other surgery, has a number of risks, besides causing discomfort, and is expensive (even if the cost is covered by insurance, she correctly reasoned that society at large pays). Yet both her primary care doctor and the surgeon, to whom she was referred, felt that she would benefit from surgery.

Different geographic areas of the Unites States have different patterns of the use of health care resources. Pamela lives in Los Angeles. Had she lived in Salt Lake City a different course of diagnosis and treatment may well have been recommended. In Salt Lake City her primary care provider would more likely have suggested she observe her symptoms for a while, prior to having an ultrasound, and note more clearly if certain activities like eating or having bowel movements were associated with her pain. She might also have looked for specific foods that may have aggravated or sparked the pains. With a conservative approach to this problem, she might have been advised to observe how the timing of her activities affected her symptoms. Since she did not have any "red flags" indicating a serious or life-threatening condition (like waking up due to the pain, fever, or weight loss) it would be safe to wait, watch carefully, and learn. Her observations could have provided additional evidence in order to make a clear diagnosis, and very likely avoid surgery. But she lived in Los Angeles. She had the surgery, and after she recovered from the operation, she found that her original, intermittent abdominal symptoms remained unchanged.

Clinical Practice Variations Across the United States

There is an atlas published by Dartmouth College that describes and quantifies the geographic differences in the way medicine is practiced. There is a significant difference in what is referred to as the "intensity" of medicine practiced in different regions of the U.S. In regions like California where a "high intensity medical practice" pattern exists, patients have more than twice the consultations with specialists, twice the number of doctor visits and double the number of laboratory procedures. They spend twice as many days in hospitals and intensive care units. They have double the number of surgeries than people in Utah, which has a more conservative ("low intensity") medical practice pattern. But Los Angeles residents do not enjoy better health or better quality of life than people in Salt Lake City.

There is evidence that shows that more care can lead to worse outcomes and worse quality of life. Both physical and psychological harm can occur from medical procedures. Not surprisingly, this atlas also shows huge differences in the costs of medical care in these two areas.

There is a misperception that more medical care equals better care and better health. Certainly in some populations that are underserved it may be true that the quality of care could be improved if more care were provided. Underuse of medical procedures, lack of modern technology, and access to medications and other treatments can be a cause of sub-standard medical care and poor health. However, quality of care can also suffer when inappropriate or ineffective care is provided. Research shows that a "high intensity" pattern in the practice of medicine is associated with lower quality of care and worse outcomes than more conservative practice patterns. *Overuse and misuse of medical resources are more likely if more medical care is provided.*

There was a study which compared health outcomes in a group that could make free medical visits with a group that had to pay part of the cost for medical visits. It found that those provided free care received about 40% more care than those with co-payments. Although more care appeared to benefit some high-risk patients with chronic medical conditions, on average the group that received free care had 40% more care but enjoyed no improvement in function or health measures than the fee-paying group. In addition, they had more pain, more worry, and a greater number of days when activity was restricted due to feeling unwell. Unfortunately, when patients have to shoulder more of the costs, they may forgo care which is both necessary and helpful as well as the care that is unnecessary. The key to a balanced and optimal approach to using health care is to engage in active, clear discussions with your doctor about which services and treatments are essential, which are discretionary, which are redundant, and the risks and benefits of all of them.

There is another study that examined the effect of "monitoring" infants who were hospitalized, but not severely ill, with the care provided in intensive care units. It was proposed that this was "safer". It was found, however, that monitored infants, in fact, did worse than those in a similar health condition that were simply provided routine care and were not monitored. These intensive care infants had more testing and more interventions because that is the practice style in the intensive care units that take care of very sick children, and the health care personnel continued this pattern of care with these not-very-ill infants as well. Intensive care units have risks that are only worth taking when clear indications exist for their use. "Monitoring" not-very-sick infants "just in case" only gives an illusion of safety.

Some people have abnormal heart rhythms that are characterized by "extra" heart beats (called "premature beats"). Studies to see if suppressing these abnormal premature beats with medications may improve a person's well-being and outcomes have shown that patients who were medicated for this purpose experienced side effects of the medicines that were unpleasant. More importantly, they had a higher death rate than patients with similar abnormal heart rhythms who were not medicated.

In a similar study, a group of patients had invasive procedures to remove chronic blockages from coronary (heart) arteries that were causing angina (chest pain from the heart). This group was compared to a group of similar patients who did not have an intervention to unclog the coronary arteries. Both groups received medications to lower the risks of future blockages. The survival rate in the two groups was the same. Some patients who had the invasive procedures had less angina after the procedures, so had less discomfort. But these procedures (and the risks, discomforts, time in the hospital and for recovery, and costs) can often be avoided by using medications first. Then, if the pain is not relieved, an invasive procedure to unclog the coronary artery could be considered electively.

Overuse is common in U.S. medicine. Antibiotics are frequently used inappropriately for viral infections, on which they have no effect, with the reasoning that they may prevent complications from a secondary bacterial infection. It is estimated that 33% of antibiotics prescribed in outpatient visits are unnecessary. This has been an important factor in the development of "superbugs", those bacteria that are becoming resistant to antibiotics. So misusing antibiotics can lead to side effects from taking them as well as to dangers to the public from loss of effectiveness of the antibiotics.

The number of stimulant prescriptions for children with a diagnosis of attention deficit disorder has skyrocketed, with experts feeling that many of these children would do better without them. Invasive studies like angiograms, insertion of stents into coronary arteries, and gastrointestinal endoscopies are often overused. Carotid artery (the artery to the brain) surgeries and hysterectomies (surgical removal of the uterus), the use of cardiac pacemakers, and putting tubes into children's ear drums have often been done without appropriate indication of need. There is much evidence that suggests that harm, not balanced by benefits, may occur from these interventions when used unnecessarily.

Even the traditional advice to have a yearly physical examination that the AMA had recommended in the past was not based on studies that looked at outcomes. People who have annual check-ups haven't been proven to have better health than those who don't. The advice was based on a *belief* that it *must* be beneficial. There is evidence that supports periodic exams and screenings, updates of immunizations, and other preventive interventions. But the optimum frequency and intensity of these periodic health appraisals vary with a patent's age and other existing health conditions. A routine physical exam each year increases the volume of medical visits and medical tests but does not result in a person living longer or having a better quality of life. Yet these routine visits to the doctor do provide an opportunity for testing whether there are risks of a disease or early warning of a disease that is not yet otherwise evident. Screening for disease is beneficial in a limited number of situations, but can be harmful if done indiscriminately. Moderation in health care, as in most aspects of life, yields the most benefits.

Incentives for More Care

There are a number of **factors and incentives that encourage an increasingly intensive pattern of medical practice**. There are incentives to use more procedures, to take more medications, and to intervene more aggressively. Physicians, hospitals, and other facilities are usually paid more when they do more. The doctor who recommends a procedure is frequently the one who performs and profits from it. Increasingly, diagnostic instruments are readily available and owned by local medical practices and groups who profit from using them. Those practices who own these instruments order more tests that use their instruments than practices that refer patients to other facilities to have the same test done. *This represents a built-in conflict of interest in the practice of medicine.* Greater intensity of practice means greater earnings.

The proliferation of malpractice suits against physicians has caused them to practice medicine more defensively. They want to protect themselves against possible charges of negligence. Therefore, if there is any question that a laboratory test may be useful at some time in the future, it is likely to be ordered right away, rather than waiting to see if it becomes really necessary. Similarly, prescribing medications earlier than absolutely needed becomes more likely. Physicians feel safer if they test at once, or intervene early, as a result of this fear of litigation.

The producers of medications, appliances, and devices, and testing equipment spend huge amounts of money marketing their products to physicians, as well as directly to consumers. We have all seen the television advertisements that assure us we will be healthier, happier, and more successful if we use their products. Now direct-to-consumer marketing of genetic testing and other laboratory tests has arrived. In some settings, the consumer can order tests without needing to involve their physician or health insurance plan. These tests are offered to the public before there has been any scientific validation of the possible risks or benefits of having these tests done. The internet is a large new source of direct marketing and sales of medical products. Most of us have received spam emails offering medications that will make us look better and feel better, even offering products to enlarge our penises! There is plenty of evidence that marketing does increase use and sales.

Although medicine is increasingly rooted in science, the practice of medicine will remain filled with uncertainty. The anxiety created by this uncertainty affects both patients and their medical providers. One way of allaying it is to "do something", which in itself can be another source of pressure to intervene or to test. The tension that uncertainty causes leads to impatience and leads to decisions aimed at diminishing this tension. "Doing something" gives us an illusion of solving the issue, even though it can sometimes result in further problems and anxiety.

Physicians have been trained to solve problems and fix the ailments that are affecting their patients. The culture of medical care is to intervene. It becomes difficult for doctors to not offer some treatment, even when it is likely to be of no benefit. Trying to fix the unfixable is counterproductive, yet is commonly observed.

"Incidentaloma"

Pamela, if you recall, had an incidental finding in her CT scan: an adrenal mass. As diagnostic testing increases and becomes increasingly sensitive, more patients will receive diagnoses that have no symptoms. If they had not had the diagnostic test, they would not have known that they had anything "abnormal". The increasingly subtle findings identified by advanced diagnostic technology create another mechanism of harm, **pseudodisease**. Pseudodisease is a disease that would never become apparent to patients during their lifetime without the diagnostic test. These incidental findings have been given a name, **incidentaloma**. This refers to an abnormality of unknown significance found in a study done for some other indication. "Oma" in medicine is a suffix used to indicate a mass or tumor, like a lymphoma is a tumor (cancer) of the lymph nodes, a lipoma is a benign fatty tumor, and a neuroma is a tumor of a nerve.

Once we know of an incidentaloma, we cannot unknow it. This can often lead to further diagnostic tests, sometimes invasive ones. This zealous pursuit is validated, occasionally, by finding a significant lesion. Yet in the case of an adrenal mass like Pamela's, only one in 4000 is found to be malignant (cancerous). The adrenal masses that have been found to be cancerous are virtually all greater than 4 centimeters (11/2 inches) in size, much bigger than Pamela's. Her incidentaloma led to more biochemical tests and will likely lead to future x-ray studies that will expose her to medical radiation, in order to monitor this mass. She now knows she has an abnormality that she had no awareness of in the past and is feeling even more vulnerable. However, 10% of people have incidental adrenal masses found in autopsy studies that caused no problems during their lifetime. As a result of the CT scan, though, Pamela will have her mass observed over time to see if this pseudodisease becomes a real disease.

Incidental findings from these new and increasingly sensitive diagnostic tests are being studied to see which of these unexpected findings actually lead to future harm. Guidelines can then be developed for rational and prudent approaches to their management. It is clear that as the increasingly sensitive technologies are developed, more incidental abnormalities will be discovered. It is important to validate each new piece of diagnostic equipment and a new test in order to use these responsibly. Yet, manufacturers are keen to promote the early use of any new test or new equipment because they profit by it. New tests and equipment are often promoted before the needed experience of their usefulness and possibilities of causing harm have been carefully examined.

False Positives and False Negatives

All medical tests can give **false positive results**, indicating the presence of a problem when there is none. They can also have **false negative results**, by not revealing the existence of an abnormality which really exists. The result is that having a test often does not resolve uncertainty, it just changes the odds. A positive result suggests that there *may* be a problem and often a confirmatory test is run.

Exercise stress tests have an 8-10% rate of false positive results. If a person has a positive exercise test suggesting coronary artery disease (blockage of the vessels in the heart) an invasive coronary angiogram may be needed to confirm this result. This invasive test has risks which include death. A cascade of testing can start with simple tests that have a minimal risk, and continue with increasingly invasive and risk-laden procedures if the initial tests indicate a possible problem. Prior to having an exercise test, or any other examination, it is important to know how the result of this test will benefit us, and what tests might follow if an uncertain result or a positive result is obtained on the initial test. It is better not to start down a path if you think, given the potential consequences, you won't want to be on it later.

An abnormal mammogram often leads to a breast biopsy. The physical discomfort of the invasive biopsy procedure is significant. Even when the biopsy is negative, evidence shows that women experience increased anxiety and distress that lasts an average of 6 months (this evidence of this increased anxiety can actually be quantified by measuring cortisol in the blood, as the level of this hormone increases as a response to stress) after a positive result is proven to be false. Studies do reveal that mammograms can prevent death from breast cancer by allowing the early discovery of a cancer that can be cured, particularly in women who are at higher than average risk. The age when it is best to start having these tests can vary, depending on family history and other factors. But studies also make clear that there are "costs" to these programs, such as false positives that lead to biopsies, and anxiety resulting from screening tests. Mammograms also expose women to radiation.

Making an informed decision about breast-cancer screening requires weighing the individual woman's risk for breast cancer (which may include age and family history as well as other personal factors) and comparing them to the risks of having the test. Don't mistake the intent here. Mammography can and does save lives. It is just important to consider who is most likely to benefit from the study, what the procedure involves, what the results might mean, and what future testing may be recommended. As always, it is best to be guided by good information and expert advice, and to make decisions based on your own preferences and values.

Beware of Men Advertising Diagnostic Tests

Irresponsible, yet all too pervasive marketing is creating a demand for people to have different types of body scans, genetic analyses, or other laboratory tests that search for risks for future diseases or for sub-clinical (not yet showing any symptoms) diseases. This type of marketing depends on creating fear in potential clients, fear that will lead to a demand for testing that will be profitable for the sellers. They create an illusion that you are being "proactive and responsible" by undergoing these tests which seems commendable. But understand that there are risks involved in any intervention or any test in medicine. A simple example of harm is that some of these scans expose us to radiation. A study from the National Cancer Institute estimated that the radiation from CT scans is the cause of 1-2% of all the cancers in the United States. As long as patients are left to rely solely on the biased advertising of manufacturers of medications, tests, and devices, and providers of unproven treatments, there will be pressures for overuse of medical care with its attendant harms.

An example illustrating how testing can lead to difficulties is provided by Mark, who is a 62-year-old man. He had read about a new test to evaluate the amount of calcium in his coronary arteries through an internet web site. The information on the web he was reviewing stated that if he had a high "calcium score" from this new computerized scan of his heart, then he had a greater chance of having a heart attack. If that were the case, he could be more disciplined in his lifestyle or perhaps take medications, and so reduce the risk. This test was offered on a fee-paying basis by a commercial vendor since it was not covered by his insurance. This is a new x-ray procedure which is being evaluated to see if the information provided can improve health care and outcomes, yet the vendor is allowed to offer this before the evaluation is complete. Mark was swayed by the marketing for this test and went to a specialized clinic offering the scan, where a doctor agreed that he might benefit from the study, and so ordered it. Mark was worried he could have "silent" heart disease such as his father had had.

The result of his scan showed that his coronary calcium score was below any level that would cause him to worry, but this scan found an abnormal nodule in his left lower lung, an area that is also viewed in the scan since it is very near the heart. He went to his primary care doctor with this information, worried that he might have lung cancer. The doctor agreed that this nodule was suspicious, and referred him to a pulmonary (lung) specialist, who recommended a needle biopsy of the nodule to make a diagnosis. When the needle was inserted into the nodule, his lung collapsed from the air released by the lung from the puncture wound, into the surrounding chest cavity. This is a known possible complication of this procedure. He was hospitalized and had a tube inserted into the chest to remove the air in his chest cavity that was not allowing his collapsed lung to expand again. After three days, his lung was healed, and he was released from the hospital. A week later he was given the "good news" that the nodule was an old scar with no sign of cancer.

This experience provoked a lot of fear and anxiety and pain lasting several months. He is now reticent to have any other diagnostic tests, fearing that he would have another unexpected finding which would lead to further tests. Anxiety from a test suggesting possible cancer can persist for six or more months after test results from further studies confirms that the abnormality was benign. While Mark paid for the initial scan, his insurance covered the subsequent tests and hospitalization.

It is important to understand what the results of a test will indicate, and what the next step would be if the result is "positive". Pamela could have asked her doctor what the ultrasound could determine, and what the next step would be if the result was positive. She would also want to know what the likelihood is that a test will give a false positive result. It is not acceptable for the answers to be ambiguous. Pamela might also have asked: "What is the risk of not having the test?" Mark, too, could have asked similar questions.

If Pamela had been advised by a Salt Lake City primary care provider to observe her symptoms before further action, she might well have felt she was "doing something" since *careful observation is as much a diagnostic test as any other sophisticated technical procedure.* And **patience is a virtue.** As Doctor William Osler stated more than a century ago, "time doth make diagnosticians of us all."

Questions to Ask

You might ask these questions to try to assess the appropriateness of tests:
- How will the results of this test affect the approach to caring for, or treating my condition?
- Will this test possibly lead to more tests, like follow-up tests or biopsies, or confirmation tests (called the "testing cascade")?
- What are the risks of this test to my health?
- What are the risks to my health of not having this test?
- Can we postpone this test and observe the condition and then reconsider?

The doctor should provide clear and specific answers to these questions. If they are not provided, it is reasonable to get a second opinion or consultation.

When a treatment is offered, you should ask these questions:
- How will this treatment or medication benefit me?
- Will it reduce my symptoms or improve the quality of my life?
- Will it help me live longer?
- Will it lower my risks for particular hazards?

Again, the doctor should provide specific answers.

Other questions to ask regarding the risks of treatments:
- What are the possible side effects or complications of this treatment or medication?
- Will it reduce my sense of well-being?
- Can it pose a risk to my health?

Chapter 6

Thieves of Autonomy

Reasons that you may be robbed of your opportunities to participate in making health care decisions include:

- The **power or authority** of the physician and medical establishment are difficult to counter.
- Your **fears and anxieties and other irrational reactions** that can occur regarding illness and health inhibit the ability to exercise your autonomy.
- The **state of being sick and dependent on others** puts you at a disadvantage.

The Power of Authority

Physicians and other clinicians are in a position of authority. They gain this from their expertise, their mastering of a body of knowledge, and their experience. Also, physicians have social power from being in an admired and respected profession. When they give information in a convincing manner (such as citing research studies or stating information in a forceful way), they increase their power and authority. In addition, the trappings of the medical establishment—the white coats, the modern technology, hospital routines, and laboratory procedures—all add to the power of the medical establishment, particularly if these settings are different from anything you are familiar with. Of course, you trust physicians to be beneficent and benevolent with their power!

After Arthur had a partial colectomy, a removal of a portion of his large bowel, for cancer of the colon, he was in a lot of pain and had difficulty sleeping. When he was awakened after finally falling asleep the night after his surgery to have his temperature and blood pressure taken, he complained that he was not being allowed to get needed sleep. The nurse explained that this was their routine and schedule, and interfering with their schedule made it difficult for them to complete their tasks. It really was for his and other patients' benefit. When he persisted in asking for some flexibility in their schedule to allow him to rest, they made their displeasure clear and said they would notify his doctor of his request. Arthur felt dependent on their care. He needed pain medication at the right time and help with his personal care, and felt at risk for complications after his operation. He was careful, after the nurses had made clear their unwillingness to change their routines, to express understanding and appreciation of their position in order to avoid being considered uncooperative. He did not want to risk any reluctance or delay in obtaining help when he might need it. He certainly did not want his doctor to see him as a problem patient!

I recall my father when he was hospitalized for a small heart attack. He was frustrated at being confined. He disliked the hospital food and was constantly interrupted by well-intentioned nursing activities. When a social worker came to visit him and asked him how he was doing, he replied: "Awful!" So she asked him what was troubling him. He said, "This isn't a vacation, you know!" It brings to mind a "Cornered" cartoon where a nurse is talking to a patient lying in a hospital bed: "Try to get some rest. I'll be in every few minutes to make sure that you don't." Yet it is unusual to question these procedures that cause a person further discomforts when they are dependent on the support from health care providers.

Patients typically want to please their doctors, to please the authority. They may try to be "good" patients by consenting to what they feel their doctors want. They may agree to proceed with an intervention they would rather not undergo—from taking medications to enduring procedures even if they are frightening or painful—rather than risk losing the doctor's good will. Even simple hospital routines like having their blood pressure, pulse, temperature, etc. taken in the middle of the night, are often readily accepted, though they may interfere with sleep and may be unnecessary. Being the authority, medical practitioners can express approval and appreciation that make patients feel accepted and that they are behaving well. This encourages continued behaviors that challenge the fine line between being compliant and losing our autonomy. It is difficult to challenge authority.

Stanley Milgram became famous by performing an experiment that demonstrated that we sometimes will do what an authority asks of us even when these actions conflict with our principles and values, or our desires. The people who participated in the study were told they were helping evaluate the role of "negative reinforcement" in learning. They were instructed to deliver an electric shock when the person playing the role of a learner answered a question incorrectly. The participants were asked to give what they thought were increasingly powerful "punishment" shocks when the learner continued to give wrong answers. More than half the participants delivered what they thought were powerful and potentially lethal shocks, in spite of the learners expressing serious distress. These controversial studies demonstrated that normal people, in following orders, were prepared to do awful things to others if commanded by a "legitimate" authority. (The electrical "shocks" in this experiment were really sham, not true shocks.)

The term *compliance* is commonly used to describe whether patients follow the plans established. A "compliant" patient is essentially a "good" or obedient patient. "Compliance" suggests that the patient is passively following the doctor's orders and that the treatment plan is not based on a therapeutic alliance or contract that is discussed and agreed upon between the patient and the physician. So even the language used is part of the process where the medical establishment imposes its authority. A term, such as "*adherence*", would be more likely to include patient participation and cooperation in formulating the plans that deal with the patient's health care concerns. The word "adherence" suggests accepting and acting on recommendations after considering them, perhaps collaborating in their formulation, and adopting them as one's own, rather than simply following orders.

Fears and Feelings When We are Sick and Dependent

Illness and discomfort make us feel vulnerable and afraid. When people are sick they may consent to advice and suggestions and routines, not because they have carefully reasoned their way to deciding in favor of them, but because they have been advised to do so by someone in authority. Sickness causes us to be more childlike in our ability to reason. We are less able to appraise relevant information critically and weigh our preferences. Sick people, being in a vulnerable position, tend to seek approval of the physician and his or her team. There is comfort in ceding control to an authority, so the patients acknowledge the physician's authority by doing what they think he wishes them to do. This can help allay feelings of vulnerability, by bringing the same sort of comfort we experienced as children when we were ill and were cared for by our parents or other loved ones.

An 80-year-old man was advised to have a "routine" exercise test as part of a periodic health appraisal, to see if he had any changes suggestive of coronary artery disease. It would have been appropriate to question the need for this procedure since he was not having any symptoms suggestive of heart problems. He had wanted to show how he was a good patient by undergoing the battery of tests recommended, however. Furthermore, he looked forward to normal test results and a "clean bill of health", which would make him feel healthy. When the results were not normal, his doctor advised him to have an urgent coronary arteriogram, an invasive study. He was told the initial test suggested that there was a narrowed artery which was at risk to close off completely. This could result in a heart attack. The precise diagnosis that an arteriogram would provide, could lead to an intervention to prevent this, or could simply show that there is no cause for concern. Again, it would have been reasonable to question this urgent test since he was feeling very well. He was now afraid about the significance of the initial results so he agreed to be hospitalized and endure this invasive procedure. This was a frightening situation, in which neither he nor his wife felt in a position to seek another opinion or to explore alternatives. It has not been shown that life expectancy or quality of life is improved by such an intervention in an 80-year-old person who has no symptoms.

Feelings, like fears and anxieties, can impair our ability to reason. We have difficulty reconciling priorities when we have powerful emotional reactions, even when we understand that these reactions are clearly irrational. This may also make us increasingly dependent on people in authority, as we attempt to reduce and control our unpleasant feelings. Fear is common when we are sick and physically dependent on others.

How does Our Ability to Think Clearly Change When We are Seriously Ill?

Serious illness is marked by losses of many normal functions in various dimensions, including the ability to reason, without which autonomy loses its meaning. A study of hospitalized patients looked at their ability to reason as they become more physically disabled (meaning that they had more difficulty in functioning independently and needing more assistance and care). All of these patients had passed the MMSE (Mini Mental Status Examination) so that they were not considered cognitively impaired and were capable of thinking clearly and to consider issues. They were given tasks to test their ability to reason.

Sicker patients were able to respond correctly to fewer tasks that required the ability to reason. So the condition of the patients or their "degree of sickness"—be it due to medications, fatigue, or physical dependence—diminished their ability to participate effectively in important decision making tasks. They had difficulty in engaging in activities that required reasoning and consideration. This resulted in their having less ability to make sound judgments about clinical decisions and physician's recommendations. They should not be considered fully capable of giving informed consent to medical procedures, nor to make a decision as to whether they should participate in a clinical study. They should also not be considered fully capable of executing other legal documents.

Thus, the innate power and authority of the medical establishment, the difficulty in reasoning that can develop when we are sick and impaired, and the emotional reactions that arise when we are dependent and in physical discomfort can, together, seriously erode or "steal" our autonomy.

In these situations, having a trusted advocate who understands our values and priorities can prove invaluable or even essential. This person can help us reason, help us consider alternative authorities to consult, and help us identify legitimate authority based on expertise and the clarity of their explanations. Such an advocate can create the space needed to seek guidance from other experts yet allow the patient to remain the final judge for him or herself. This advocate can be a family member, a trusted professional, or a friend. It is a relationship with a fundamental responsibility to help a patient assert or reassert his or her authentic autonomy.

Section 3

Aging and Health Care

Aging, the process of becoming older, represents the accumulation of changes in a human being over time. In the first two or three decades of our life, we develop skills and abilities. It is a period of physical and mental and intellectual growth as we mature. During this time, the biological process of renewal allows this growth, without evident declines in our ability to respond to stresses. After these early years, the impact of the aging process becomes manifest. Once we are over 60 to 65 years old, the consequences of the aging process become increasingly noticeable. Injuries (head injuries seen in wars or during sporting activities for example) or chronic illnesses (diabetes for example), as well as lifestyle choices (smoking for example), can accelerate this process.

Advancements in sanitation and public health and medical science have increased life expectancy by more than 80% over the last century. As a result, there are many more senior citizens now living with the results of these changes due to living to an advanced age. The numbers of people 65-and-older jumped 15.1 percent between 2000 and 2010, compared with a 9.7% increase for the total U.S. population. The 41 million people age 65 and older now make up 15% of the total population in the United States compared with 12.4% in 2000 and 4.1 percent in 1900. Older people have priorities particular to their demographic group, which influence their preferences and choices in the approach to health care. The desire to remain engaged with their families and in their communities and to live independently as long as possible is commonly described.

There now is a primary medical care specialty for older adults called *Geriatrics* that focuses on the particular health care needs of the elderly. The aged body is different physiologically from the younger adult body, and during old age, the decline of various organ systems becomes evident. Geriatricians use their understanding of these differences in providing medical care for elders. Functional abilities, independence and the quality of life are of great concern to geriatricians and their patients.

Exercising autonomy as an ethical principle continues to offer better outcomes for individuals and society throughout our lifetimes. In this section, we examine the perspectives and influences that aging may offer in making informed choices regarding our health care. We can plan to exercise our autonomy in anticipation of losing our capacity to make or express our choices. **Advance Directives** are the legal documents that extend your ability to make health care choices into the future, and we will explore these. As we near death the choices we make (or have already made and documented) can have an important and lasting impact on your loved ones. We will consider the choices available to us as our life is ending.

Chapter 7
Aging and Health Care Choices
Preparing to go Slow

Continuing with the principle of autonomy, as you participate in making health care decisions for yourself and your loved ones, this chapter discusses how getting older may influence the informed choices you will make. Aging is inevitable. Becoming old is the result of this process. So aging is not a judgment or a criticism. It is part of being alive. Understanding the nature of the aging process and the results of becoming old can help us consider how this can be a factor in our approaches to health care decisions.

My intention in using "*Preparing to Go Slow*" as a subtitle for this chapter is twofold. First, by "preparing" I do not mean passively waiting or expecting to be slowing down. Preparing requires an active effort, an intention you must put energy and thought and work into. And with "to go slow", I am (knowing that it is incorrect grammar) invoking a concept gaining attention in geriatric medicine, and that is "*slow medicine*" which promotes not slowing down physically but paying attention to our basic needs and moving at the "right speed".

Integrated into this chapter are perspectives and ideas from writings and conversations of three physicians I respect, along with my own thoughts:

Atul Gawande particularly from his 2014 book, **Being Mortal**;

Ezekiel Emanuel, particularly from a provocative article in the **Atlantic** in 2014;

Dennis McCullough who articulated the philosophy of *Slow Medicine*.

Their ideas, while framed from different perspectives, share common concerns and philosophies about the last portion of our life, including our losses of capacities and functions as we age, the transition from independence to dependence, and finally how our lives end—and how the health care choices we make can have an important impact on our experience and a lasting impact on those we love.

Atul Gawande is a highly respected writer and thinker about the health care system. He has written books and articles that have had an influence on the health care establishment as well as on governmental policies. I really value his understanding of the relationships between doctors and patients, and how each impacts the other. He is aware of the pressure that doctors feel to intervene and fix problems, and that patients feel to follow their advice.

In his 2014 book, **Being Mortal,** he describes his view that modern scientific advances have turned the process of aging and dying into medical experiences, to be intervened with and managed by health care professionals.

Aging is not a medical diagnosis, it is normal. Death is inevitable. Neither should be considered a defeat. We become victims if we are not clear that this is the normal life cycle. We can fall into medical traps we never wanted or expected. The more we medicalize aging and dying, the more we intervene with testing and procedures, the more likely we are to end up institutionalized, hospitalized—possibly in intensive care units—that cut us off from our communities, families and everything we value.

In the chapter called "**Things fall Apart**" Gawande discusses the normal aging process. For example, our bones lose calcium, becoming weaker. Our arteries gain calcium and become stiffer. We lose muscle and hence strength. Our lungs get stiffer; it gradually becomes harder to fill them with air, and the volume of air in each breath decreases. Our heart gets stiffer making it harder to fill with blood and the pumping is less efficient, so we tire faster and get short of breath more easily. Our joints get stiffer making it harder to move. Our nerves lose insulation, so they conduct more poorly and we lose some sensation. Our fine motor control is poorer, making it more difficult to use zippers or to put on jewelry. Our balance gets worse, we get less steady. It gets harder to stand up from a low chair. Our brains process ideas and words more slowly, so we cannot make the quick comeback. Sometimes we cannot remember a word or name, even though we know they are in our mind yet cannot bring them up. We gradually lose our memory.

The body declines with age. It creeps up on us. We are born with great redundancy. We have two lungs when we could get along fine with one, particularly in our earlier years; we have two kidneys, our liver is "over" capable, and we need only a small portion of the full capacity of our brain in our first few decades. All our other systems also have excess capacity when we are young. But losses occurring randomly over decades accumulate until they overcome this built in extra capacity or redundancy of our systems, and the losses become more noticeable. Often this is a gradual process, but sometimes these decreases in capacities are made evident by a sudden event, such as a fall, a stroke, an illness, a vehicle accident, and we do not fully recover.

We fall apart! Our performance of every-day tasks and activities become progressively less and less efficient and less and less effective. We are getting older.

Technological advances have improved our health and well-being. In 1900 life expectancy in the U.S. at birth was 47 years. By 1960 it had reached 69.7 years. Most of this gain was due to lowering the number of premature deaths with civil engineering advances which improved sanitation and thus reduced infectious diseases. Also, medical advances like vaccinations and antibiotics prevented deaths of vulnerable younger individuals, as well as better prenatal care, which lowered the number of deaths of mothers giving birth and their infants. This had a large impact on life expectancy. If a life is saved at 1 or 2 years of age, they now may live another 75 years which has a potent influence on the average life expectancy. From 1960 to 2015, life expectancy has increased another 12.3 years. These gains are mainly due to a reduction in smoking, better medications for vascular disease prevention, and controlling hypertension. So in the last 55 years, we have prevented early deaths of mature adults. The result is that we now have a large elderly population. There were more than 18 million people in the United States in 2015 over 75 years old.

This increase in the population of people in their senior years who have accumulated those losses in capacity results in an increase in the number of people who live years of their lives with decreased function, and an increase in the number of years they live with disabilities. Yet the focus of medical care has remained to extend life rather than the retention of the abilities that keep us functioning well. This commonly continues even when we are very old and life extension can realistically not add much time. Life extension then can become extending a life of dependence and inability to be engaged actively in the world.

Gawande wants the focus of medical care for the elderly to support quality of life, to lower the ravages of diseases. The main goal should be to retain the ability to be active and socially engaged and independent. One example of such a medical advance that improves the quality of life is joint replacement surgery. When arthritis causes pain in walking and moving, we now have the capacity to replace some damaged joints with artificial ones. That can relieve pain and improve our functional abilities and improve the quality of life.

Ezekiel Emanuel shares a similar view to Gawande's in his article in the *Atlantic* but from a more provocative perspective. He is an oncologist and bioethicist at the University of Pennsylvania School of Medicine. He has written a number of books and articles, is a respected academic, and was an advisor to President Obama in his first term of office.

The article I am referring to, published in October of 2014, is titled **"Why I Hope to Die at 75."**

Emanuel was 57 when it was published. Perhaps as he nears the age of his hopes he may change his opinion about this chosen age. But he feels quite certain about the philosophy he describes in the article. As an academic, he uses a lot of medical and public health evidence to support his argument.

He describes how over the last 50 years, health care has **not slowed the process of aging so much as it has slowed the process of dying**. Death after 75 usually is the result of a chronic illness which gradually progresses over time, such as vascular disease or degenerative diseases including dementia, or cancer.

He acknowledges that there are a number of remarkable elderly individuals who continue to live full lives and contribute to their communities and society at large. They continue to enjoy good physical and mental health. But they are the exception. He does not want to test the odds of being the exception. By definition, few of us can be an exception. Yet we are urged to make medical decisions by the health care system as if we will be that special case. But as the aging process is a natural and relentless process, even when we beat overwhelming odds, it is only for a brief period of time.

For example, chemotherapy after 75 is offered for many cancers yet does not statistically prolong life. There are rare exceptions. There are **no** exceptions to the side effects of chemotherapy, these are guaranteed. Frequently these side effects leave people dependent and disabled for extended periods of time, possibly until they die of the disease or the treatment, or from another condition that may have been worsened by the treatment. In seeking to be the exception, the odds are against us. The probability of worsening our life is much greater than that of significantly extending it.

That is a similar concern that Gawande shares with us. He describes the survival curve of people diagnosed with mortal conditions as having a long but slender tail to the right (graph below). This means that rare individuals do survive for a long time after being given a diagnosis of a likely mortal illness. Yet it is common to think we will be the one to be that long tail—and the medical establishment encourages doctors and patients to think this way. If you choose to look for this tail, you at least need to prepare for the probable consequences.

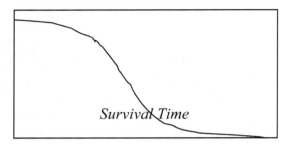

Survival Curve with Tail

So Emanuel has decided, on a practical level, in order to avoid the emotional and physical restrictions and discomforts, as well as the financial burdens imposed by aging, that he will not slow the dying process. He does not want to impose this burden on his family. His choice of a specific date gives him a clear delineation on when he will change his approach to his own health care. He feels he can avoid the traps and fuzziness in making decisions by having a clearly defined date. He will not need to ask, "Is this the right time to stop interventions?"

He says at 75 he will not go to the doctor unless there is a good reason, such as relieving discomfort or pain. He will not have tests or treatments that are aimed towards extending his life, only those that will aid the in the quality of his life. He will refuse any preventive tests or screening. He will refuse any cardiac stress tests, any cancer screening, and he will have no treatments for cancer. He will refuse a pacemaker, valve replacement, defibrillators, or dialysis.

He will be sure to have his advance directives up to date and to have an active **Do Not Resuscitate** order in place.

He is aware that standard medical care continues to offer treatments and interventions that sacrifice the quality of our existence now for gaining future time. And when we are elderly, future time is not really available.

The medical culture is built around the long tail suggesting we are all potentially the long survivors, which becomes the equivalent of buying lottery tickets. You could be the winner. It becomes an emotional bias that is difficult to resist and be clear about. Gawande describes the pressure he feels as a physician to do something, even when it is futile and counterproductive, possibly causing pain and suffering.

The diagnosis and approach to cancer is one example of this process. It has been observed that oncologists overestimate survival time for their patients, often five-fold (an average of 530% overestimation of time left to live before death from the cancer), they overestimate the curability of cancers, and 40% of oncologists admit to offering treatments that **they know** will not be effective. This miscalibration happens in many other chronic health conditions. I greatly appreciate Gawande's understanding of the pressure health care providers feel to fix that which is unfixable. That is our training, the direction that medical education gives to physicians.

So we wait for the doctor to tell us there is nothing more that can be done. But there is always something they can do!

There are Alternatives

There are published studies that illustrate other options and their outcomes.

One study looked at the impact of a hospice program, where attention is given to the quality of life, compared with routine care from primary care physicians and specialists ("usual care"), where more emphasis is placed on prolonging life. There were 4,493 individuals in this study with conditions that left them with less than three years of life expectancy. Half received hospice care and the other half had usual care. Patients with advanced breast cancer, prostate cancer, and colon cancer, showed no difference in survival between the two groups. In patients with pancreatic cancer, the group receiving hospice care lived 3 more weeks than those in the usual care group. Those with lung cancer lived 6 more weeks, and those with congestive heart failure lived 3 more months with hospice support than those in the routine and specialist care group. And the patients in a hospice program had less chemotherapy, fewer visits to the emergency rooms, were hospitalized less, spent fewer days in the intensive care unit, and more frequently died at home.

The conclusion in this study was that you live better and longer when you stop trying to live longer!

Another study published in 2010 in the **New England Journal of Medicine** was a prospective study (a study that follows the patients over time to observe the impact of the management of their disease) of 151 patients with advanced non-small cell lung cancer (the most common type of lung cancer). All patients had the usual care from oncologists, but one-half was also given additional care from palliative care specialists.

Palliative care is a specialty that is aimed at the relief of pain and discomfort with no intention to cure and encourages patients to be involved in making their own medical decisions (See Chapter 8).

The results were that those in the group who received palliative care plus care from oncologists chose to have less aggressive treatments such as chemotherapy. They spent fewer days in the hospital and fewer days in the intensive care unit than the group that received care only from cancer specialists. They suffered less pain. And in measures of quality of life and depression, they scored much better. And they lived 25% longer on average, 11.6 months as opposed to 8.9 months in the group under the care of the oncologists only.

So those who focused on quality of life achieved better emotional states, spent less time feeling poorly, less time in the hospital, and lived longer, and their death was more peaceful.

Slow Medicine

Dennis McCullough was a geriatrician and professor at Dartmouth College School of Medicine. He described his concept of *Slow Medicine* in his book, **My Mother, Your Mother,** which was based on his own experiences during the final years of his Mother's life. I was fortunate to have had the opportunity to explore his perspectives personally with him.

Some background—in 1986 a man named Carlo Petrini started a protest against the opening of a new McDonald's in Piazza de Spagna, Rome. He said he wanted an *alternative to fast food; he wanted what he called **Slow Food**.* The concept caught on and became an international movement, promoting the idea that slow food represented regional and local food, produced in sustainable ways, picked when it is ripe and ready to be used. The selection of products would vary according to the seasons, and we would benefit by waiting for the produce to be ready for consumption. This results in improved nutritional quality and better flavors. It also decreases the waste of time and fuel spent in transportation and storage.

The *slow food* movement led to the development of other *slow movements*. The concept spread to slow travel, slow tourism, slow design, slow publishing, and slow cities. In 1999 the "*The World Institute of Slowness*" was established as a think tank in Norway. They describe the idea of a **slow planet.** (You can see all it entails in their web site, *theworldinstituteofslowness.com*.) The philosophy for a slow planet was described as follows:

*Faster is not always better. "Slow" means doing things at the **right** speed. Savoring rather than counting was preferred. Quality over quantity was promoted.*

As everything is changing, we feel we need to speed up just to hang on, to multitask. ***But our basic needs do not change.*** **The slow planet recognizes this and pays attention.** The slow planet is good for individuals and protects the environment. It reduces waste and reduces carbon emissions. It promotes having ample time and space for careful observation and contemplation. Details can be explored, appreciated and understood. We can stop and smell the roses!

In the medical establishment, the preference of many administrators and doctors is for "efficiency". Rather than spending valuable time listening and understanding, we shunt patients off for tests and procedures, as long as they are covered by insurance. Insurances pay much more for these tests and procedures than time spent talking and listening, what can be called **the soft technology of medicine**. And more patients can be seen. The current practice of medicine is best at managing crises, performing elective procedures and specialty care, using the latest technological developments. But for the management of common conditions that are seen in aging, those slow-moving diseases that require support done by one-on-one discussions of details for their best management, medicine is not doing so well.

McCullough sums it up: "The vast machinery of modern medicine, which can heroically save a premature baby, when visited upon an equally vulnerable and failing grandmother, may not save her life as much as tortuously and inhumanely complicate her dying." Some elderly patients are therefore subjected to what is called "death by intensive care".

No one seems to know how to apply the brakes to fast medicine. What he proposes in "slow medicine" is for families, friends, and neighbors to team up with health care providers and visiting nurses, to meet the basic needs, avoid unnecessary care, and to attend to the day to day needs of the elderly by offering emotional support, social stimulation, better nutrition, and making moving, sleeping, and everyday tasks easier. Care givers will also offer support and assistance to do all the transactions necessary in everyday life. The primary goal is to help these patients stay in their homes and to remain as independent as possible. The quality of life is the priority.

There is evidence for the benefits of slow medicine. In one study of 568 patients over 70 who were considered at risk for institutionalization due to chronic health conditions or mild losses of mental capacities, half were assigned to a geriatric team which paid attention to small issues like foot care, skin care, nutrition, simplifying how medicines are taken, and increasing social activity. Team members went periodically to the patient's homes. They practiced slow medicine. The other half had the usual care offered by their primary care providers. All were followed for 18 months.

The results revealed that 10% of each group died, so no difference was observed in mortality over the 18 months of the study. However, among the patients with the geriatric team, there was 25% less disability, 25% lower depression scores, and 40% less need for home-care support.

More independence and better quality of life in the Slow Medicine Group!

Another trial offered hospice services concurrent with the usual care—so patients did not give up curative treatments for any serious conditions, and hospice was not limited to those nearing death. During home visits, hospice nurses paid attention to personal care advice and to the small daily issues that keep arising such as nutrition, skin care, accident prevention, and to social concerns for the patient and other family members. The others had only the usual care. Those in the combined care groups had less than half the visits to emergency rooms and a greater than two-thirds reduction in time spent in ICUs and hospitals. There was no difference in longevity during two years of follow-up.

Again, there was a lower use of medical resources, less time spent in hospital care, and better quality of life among the patients offered the slow medicine program. The length of life was the same.

Dartmouth College publishes an atlas of the U.S. using Medicare claims data that describes the geographic differences in the way medicine is practiced. There is a significant variation in what is referred to as the "intensity" of medicine practiced in different parts of the country.

In this atlas, some areas such as Southern California and Florida are classified as having a high intensity of medical practice. Senior citizens in these areas have more than twice the number of visits to doctors and specialists, more than twice the number of CT scans, MRIs, stress tests, and lab tests than those in Utah, which is classified as an area of low intensity of medical care for senior citizens. In high-intensity areas, seniors spend twice as many days in a hospital and in intensive care units, have twice the number of surgeries than do people of the same age in Utah. But they do not have improved outcomes or live longer.

There are regional cultures that result in these differences in the practice of medicine. These differences are also seen between nations, where different approaches to health care and the payment for medical care are chosen. This means that the incentives for choosing interventions and tests and treatments are different. In all developed nations, however, there are times when the health services and medical interventions provided can be counterproductive. Reform within the larger medical system in the United States seems improbable. So how can you slow down the medical care **you** receive?

Be Prepared!

There are strategies that can enhance your opportunities to be heard and your priorities to be respected. These require planning and preparing for the visits, and are described in chapter 4, **Going to the Doctor**.

Remember, visits to a doctor have limited time allotments to cover concerns and complete the required documentation. The opportunity to state your full agenda in medical visits is limited, with an observation that in only 8% of visits was this completed. Sometimes the doctor focuses on what he feels is the purpose of the visit only. At other times, while you are beginning to describe the reasons for your visit, something in that description catches the physician's attention and he *redirects* all the attention to this problem. This redirection was observed to happen in an average of 23.1 seconds in one study of physician styles of practice. This is fast!

And fast speed also adds to your difficulties in understanding and remembering the explanations, plans, and instructions. It is accepted that patients remember 50% or less of their instructions immediately after the visit. Instructions may be difficult to understand. Can you remember how many times a day a pill should be taken, for how many days, on an empty stomach or with food?

Improving the chances that your visit will cover your concerns and be more fruitful requires preparation. Being passive and just hoping that the doctor will know what really needs to be addressed and how to take care of these needs is just wishful thinking. Yet our own anxieties and desires to be a good patient add to the chances we will be unable to make the visit truly successful.

Your preparation for the visit should begin by first thinking of your goals for the visit ahead of time and list them in writing days before the visit. Having your list with you during your visit improves the chances to have all your items considered. It is also wise to review your priorities before the visit, so if your doctor suggests diagnostic tests, a stress test or a cancer screen, an MRI, or sleep study—those that Atul Gawande describes as frequently used unnecessarily in the elderly population—you can be ready to ask how will the results of these tests be used in the management of your care? Will they be helpful in meeting what you see as your goals? What are the chances the tests will give false positive information and lead to a more intrusive testing cascade going forward? "Do you feel that this test or this treatment will be truly helpful for me?"

You should also be prepared to tell your providers that you will need time to consider their suggestions. Processing the recommendations at home removes distractions we face when we are in the doctor's office. Slowing the process down allows you to carefully consider your reactions.

Having someone accompany you is another way of lessening the intensity of feelings around the medical visit. The **support** provided by having a companion can be significant. When the issues are complex or overwhelming, going to a visit with a companion or advocate offers great advantages. This is particularly the case when the visit is due to an unexpected or urgent concern, or when you are in discomfort.

Your feelings when you are in pain or afraid, or even simply surprised by the news, can make it difficult to pay full attention to the doctor. It is easy, in these cases, to forget simple instructions, and it can make it difficult to ask for the clarifications you may need to follow the treatment plan. A companion can help assure you have the time and space you need to settle down and gain perspective on the situation. They can ask questions for you.

Having a clear understanding of the plans for diagnostic testing and treatment is important. It increases the likelihood you will follow the recommendations. Writing the information down as it is given can reduce the chance of not remembering it later. The note taker can be either you or someone who accompanies you.

What comes after the visit? How and when can you expect results? How will you be informed? A written list of these questions so you can refer to them before the visit ends can remind you to ask them.

Preparing for the medical visit, having help in remembering and understanding the explanation, being accompanied and supported, and keeping notes are useful tools that make it more likely you will be able to adhere to the program recommended and get the most benefit out of the health care you receive.

A final point, we can never really know how much longer we have left to live, but we only die once. Having a conversation with your family and your doctor about your end-of-life choices should not wait. It has been shown that people who had such a conversation with their doctor were more likely to die in peace and in some control of their situation. They spared their families anguish. There are published reports that people who had conversations with the health care provider about their end of life preferences suffered less pain, were less likely to be hospitalized, and had better final interactions with their family members. In addition, six months after the death, the close family members were significantly less likely to suffer from depression.

Chapter 8

Choices as the End of Life Approaches

Death is inevitable. For most people, it results from conditions and diseases that are managed over weeks or months, sometimes years. But even after someone is given a diagnosis of a mortal condition, the remaining months, weeks or days of life can still be rich and fulfilling. As the end of life approaches the quality of life is best preserved by harmonizing social, spiritual, psychological, and health care support.

Many people, upon understanding they have a terminal condition, speak of a deepening moment-to-moment sense of life and connection to the people who matter most to them. They feel that the time remaining is precious and want to share it with those they love. The involvement of the family and friends as well as those groups and communities that have been meaningful for the patient and their loved ones can contribute to this *harmony of care* by providing attention, assistance, and support. Spending time with a person as the end of their life approaches can be a fulfilling spiritual and emotional experience.

These are times when family and friends can interact with love and express deeply felt emotions. Stories and memories can be shared. Brothers and sisters, children, grandchildren, and others can "make up for lost time", perhaps heal old wounds. In the final month of his life, my father told me stories of his experiences as a younger man that he had never shared before. He clearly had an ease and interest not felt before in sharing these old memories. It left me with a broader understanding of his life. It provides an enduring sweet and warm memory of him, and our time together in those final days before his death.

These last days of life can be an opportunity for understanding and resolution. It can be a time when expressions of love and intimate sharing become a priority over more material or mundane concerns. Oliver Sacks, the well-known neurologist, and best-selling author, on learning he had terminal cancer wrote:

"Over the last few days, I have been able to see my life as from a great altitude, as a sort of landscape, and with a deepening sense of connection of all its parts. This does not mean I am finished with life.

"On the contrary, I feel intensely alive, and I want and hope in the remaining time to deepen my friendships, to say farewell to those I love...and to achieve new levels of understanding and insight.

"This will involve audacity, clarity and plain speaking. But there will be time, too, for fun.

"I feel a sudden clear focus and perspective."

The patient and the family can make choices for the support that will best provide an opportunity to spend this valuable time together. The preferences of the patient and the family in addition to the condition of the person nearing death can influence greatly how this final part of life is experienced. Pain, cognitive abilities, alertness, and other physical and emotional conditions will likely influence the choices that are made as a person nears their death.

To maximize the opportunities of having rich experiences at the end of life with family members, partners, and other significant people it is important that the patient is in an environment that is welcoming and accepting of their particular values and identities. A leader in the LGBTQ (lesbian, gay, bisexual, transgender, and queer) community told me that fellow members express particular concerns about judgment or condemnation of their orientations and identities. These can cause fear, tension, or sadness and inhibit open interactions. This may lead to isolation and make it difficult to share feelings and concerns openly. These fears may cause a patient to refuse services and support that can provide an environment that is caring and dignified at the end of life.

Service providers and staff from facilities that have the cultural competence to understand diverse backgrounds and interests, increase the opportunity for maximizing the quality of time remaining in a person's life. Religious beliefs, ethnic identity, sexual orientation, gender identity, and other culturally based values and experiences need to be honored and accepted to achieve a true harmony with all areas of a patient's care. This may require support from their own community in making sure these sensitive needs are respected. There are organizations that provide training in particular cultural competences and can provide information about suitably trained providers. An example of this for the LGBTQ community is SAGE (Services and Advocacy for Gay, Lesbian, Bisexual and Transgender Elders; http://sageusa.care/). There are other organizations that offer support for particular ethnic and religious groups.

Frequently there is a sort of fog that descends on patients, their families, and care providers when they are in this challenging period near the end of life. There is often a lack of clarity regarding the trajectory of the medical condition or illness and what the benefits and burdens that any intervention may bring. Obtaining support and advice from care givers and community members who have experience of this important period can be invaluable.

You have choices as the end of life approaches. Your care and support may be done at home or in another facility. You can choose to stop all life-sustaining treatments. This means you can discontinue any treatment already in place, such as a feeding tube, medications, breathing assistance, chemotherapy, antibiotics, dialysis, blood transfusions, etc. You can ask that a pacemaker be turned off. You can decide not to initiate new treatments. *This does not mean medications or treatments that can control pain or treat other discomforts are eliminated.*

People want to be in control of decisions about their own care. Yet frequently at the end of life, there are numerous factors that can work against realizing this. Many people nearing the end of life are no longer sufficiently alert or may have physical and cognitive impairments that make it difficult to express their choices. It may be difficult to recognize that the end of life is approaching. It is important to have conversations about end-of-life choices with health care providers, family, and a chosen advocate well in advance. Yet such discussions frequently do not take place because we wait for the doctor or the family members to initiate them. Even when they do take place, there can be confusion, or it may be emotionally difficult to invoke any preferences or decisions that had been discussed previously. Advance Directives and other care planning choices made earlier may need to be reviewed at this time by the patient and family members and the chosen person to be in charge of invoking the decisions (see Chapter 9).

Stopping treatments or asking to be discharged from a hospital or another institution is your right, yet may be met with resistance. This reluctance to end support and treatment that prolongs life is understandable. Hospitals and other such establishments were founded to help heal, to treat disease, and to prolong life. There is also an interest to make certain that the placement and resolution for a patient in their care is reasonable, safe, and comfortable. This can delay implementing the choices the patient and the family insist on. Sometimes there are religious beliefs that enter into this resistance. So stopping treatments or leaving a facility may feel to those service providers, based on their training and experience, not to be following the safest course.

There are also financial incentives in medical establishments for continuing treatments. Nowadays, about 25-30% of all Medicare outlays are for care in the last year of beneficiaries' lives. This means that people nearing death are typically having medical interventions, often in hospitals and intensive care units that are costly. These interventions, by definition, do not prevent death, and may deny the person's opportunities to be with their loved ones and share this important time of a person's life. This trend has been noted for several decades and is felt to be due to the medicalization of the dying process when intervening becomes futile and counterproductive.

At times this resistance to a patient's wishes is framed in a strong, authoritative, even threatening tone. There may be threats of nonpayment from insurance, or of not supporting ongoing and essential needs for comfort care if the choice taken is against the medical care giver's advice. Insurance companies have not stopped payments in these circumstances, however, and health care providers may not simply abandon their patients. You will need to be clear, firm, and assertive about your decisions. Your choices, while stated in a convincing form, can still be framed with gratitude for the concern the health care providers have shown, and let them know you are not refusing further palliative or other support from them as it becomes necessary.

Other choices that will be discussed in this chapter include hospice care, palliative care, terminal sedation, and patient-controlled death.

Hospice

Hospice is a medical service that specializes in providing care for the dying. Hospice care focuses on the palliation of a terminally or seriously ill person's pain and discomfort. This includes physical symptoms and emotional and spiritual needs. Hospice care also involves assisting the patients' family members. They help them provide the care and support needed to keep the patient at home and help them cope with the difficulties of a loved one nearing death. Assistance in bathing, feeding, skin care, and other daily needs can be provided. Bereavement support is also part of Hospice care, so family members are supported even after their loved one dies. There are also some inpatient hospital facilities that provide hospice care. Hospice care is usually instituted when there is an acceptance that the end of life is near and that aggressive curative treatments are not being considered. When a person reaches the point that additional medical treatments are counterproductive, hospice can offer the hope of a comfortable and dignified death.

In the United States, Medicare, Medicaid, and other health insurance providers cover care by hospice providers when the patient has a medical condition with a terminal prognosis diagnosed by a physician who certifies that their life expectancy is less than 6 months. Once hospice care is instituted, it can continue indefinitely until the patient dies (even if the person lives more than 6 months). Sometimes a person recovers and "graduates" out of hospice. It can always be reinstituted in the future. This saves money because curative procedures including emergency room visits and hospitalizations are avoided. This, in turn, avoids the emotional trauma of unnecessary medical interventions and trips to health care facilities. The Medicare hospice benefits include pharmaceuticals and supplies, medical equipment, 24-hour access to care, and support for loved ones following a death.

Historically, "hospitality" for the ill and dying, particularly for the poor was provided by religious organizations. This was for the care of persons with illnesses for which no cure was available such as Tuberculosis. The attention included the basic needs such as room and board, help in daily living activities, as well as spiritual and emotional support. The growth of the hospice movement in the last century, starting with volunteers and religious orders providing services has grown internationally. It is now an established medical specialty with physicians, nurses, social workers and other trained personnel providing the services.

Each year, more than 1.5 million Americans receive hospice services. It is common for hospice care to be requested very late, often in the last few days of life. 35% of people who have hospice care don't even receive one week of the service. People nearing the end of life and their families express great appreciation for the care of hospice and commonly state they should have instituted this much earlier. It can be difficult to admit that an individual's disease has progressed so much that additional treatment is impractical and ineffective, but caregivers and their families can lose out on irrecoverable time with a dying loved one if they wait too long to seek hospice care.

Palliative Care

Palliative care is a medical specialty that focuses on providing relief of symptoms such as pain and other discomforts, as well as the stress of a serious illness. These specialists have no intention to seek a cure. The goal is to improve the quality of life for both the patient and their family. Palliative care teams are made up of doctors, nurses, and other professional medical caregivers, often initiated at the facility where a patient will have first received treatment for their illness. These professionals will administer or oversee most of the ongoing comfort care patients receive. Palliative care teams make an effort to learn what the individual wishes and prefers. They develop relationships with the patients and their families and urge them to participate in making health care decisions.

Hospice care and palliative care are very similar when it comes to the most important issue for dying people, *care*. Many people have heard of hospice care and have a general idea of what services hospice provides. What they don't know or what may become confusing is that hospice provides "palliative care".

Palliative care is both a method of administering "comfort" care and increasingly, uses established protocols to relieve pain and discomfort offered commonly by hospitals. As adjuncts or supplements to some of the more "traditional" care options, both hospice and palliative care protocols offer a combined approach where medications, day-to-day care, equipment, bereavement counseling, and symptom treatment are administered through a single program. Where palliative care programs and hospice care programs differ is in the location, timing, payment, and eligibility for services.

While palliative care can be administered in the home, it is most common to receive palliative care in an institution such as a hospital, extended care facility, or nursing home that supports palliative care teams. There are no time restrictions. Palliative care can be received by patients at any time and at any stage of illness whether it is terminal or not.

Since this service will generally be initiated through a hospital or regular medical provider, it will likely be covered by regular medical insurance. Since there are no time limits on when you can receive palliative care, it acts to fill the gap for patients who want and need comfort at any time during their illness, regardless if the onset was recent, or a chronic or terminal disease. With palliative care, there is no expectation that life-prolonging therapies will be avoided. It is appropriate for patients of any age and at any stage of a serious illness. It can be provided along with curative treatment. The palliative care team may work together with a patient's other doctors to provide that extra layer of support.

There are studies that have examined the quality of care at the end of life. Family assessments of the quality of care were significantly higher when patients had palliative care consultations during the last weeks or months of their lives. The highest reported quality of care was when patients had palliative or hospice care.

Terminal Sedation

There is much interest in the maintenance of dignity during the final days or hours of a person's life. It is common for people to express the desire to have some control over how and when they will die. Some people even request help in dying, and there are political movements towards empowering individuals to make these decisions. The states of Oregon, Washington, Vermont, and California have passed so-called "Death with Dignity" laws which set up a strictly regulated method of speeding one's death. An individual who is in the last six months of life as verified by physicians, and who is not mentally ill, can request and receive medications that will cause their death. Montana's Supreme Court decided that individuals in Montana have the right decide to hasten their death in particular situations. In Oregon, where the law has been in effect since 1997, from 40 to 50 persons speed their deaths each year by taking the lethal prescription. Similar laws exist in Holland, Belgium, Switzerland, Luxemburg, and now in Canada.

Dr. Jack Kevorkian publicly championed a terminally ill patient's right to die via euthanasia and claims to have assisted over 120 patients to that end. Because of his videotaped and publicized activities in assisting patients to die outside the context of legal safeguards, he was sentenced to prison for second-degree murder in 1999. The controversial actions of Kevorkian, as well as the "Death with Dignity" laws and the controversies around the ethics of assisting patients to die, have increased the interest in having strategies that ease discomfort in the final moments of life, but are not aimed at speeding death. This has led to substantial improvements in palliative care.

According to the Council on Ethical and Judicial Affairs of the American Medical Association (AMA), it is unethical to hasten death or to help patients die. It is also illegal to administer medications with the purpose of helping a person to die outside a specific legal protocol where it exists. In most states, there is no legal method to provide a patient with a method to commit suicide, so this option is not one that you can reasonably request under the principle of autonomy, except in those states with the legal protocols for this. Even in states with existing "Death with Dignity" laws, not all doctors will agree to offer such services in agreement with those influential organizations that express ethical concerns.

Terminal sedation (also known as **palliative** sedation) is the practice of giving a patient sedative medication that will induce sleep or unconsciousness until such time as death occurs as a result of the underlying illness or disease. Usually, the sedative is given by intravenous or subcutaneous injection. This is considered as a last resort when there is an insufficient response to medications that would otherwise ease suffering. There is the risk of a "double effect" of terminal sedation. Although the intention is to relieve suffering, administering the sedatives may contribute to an earlier death.

An example of this may be seen in the following story. Darcy had metastatic cancer of his salivary gland. His tumors were growing in his throat and neck affecting his ability to breathe and swallow. They were not responding to any treatments to slow their growth, and he was experiencing increasing levels of pain and shortness of breath. He was under the care of a hospice program with the aim of making him as comfortable and as alert as possible during the remaining days of his life. He made it clear that he wanted the pain to be controlled even if it meant sacrificing alertness.

On the last day of his life, after having breakfast with his family, he began experiencing increasing and unbearable pain. The hospice nurse during her regular visit that day talked privately with him about the loss of awareness that would come if his pain were to be relieved with additional medications, and that he would probably never regain awareness. He accepted this eventuality. He met with each of his family members present to say goodbye, then the medication was administered. He died peacefully 12 hours later, with his family by his side.

In 2008, the AMA's council on Ethical and Judicial Affairs approved as ethical the practice of palliative sedation. This practice is now legal in the United States and in many European countries (it is not legal in some countries) under legal safeguards that include counseling and informed consent. It makes it easier for the patient to die in comfort and dignity, knowing that relief will be available. It does not causally contribute to death. It constitutes help *in dying* and not help *to die*.

Considering the possibility of being in severe distress during the final period of life, it is important that you make clear your wishes for the relief of suffering even if it sacrifices your alertness. This can be done with your health care providers, with hospice personnel if they are involved in this final period of your life, and with the person you have chosen in your Durable Power of Attorney for Health Care (chapter 9).

Patient Controlled Death

Another end-of-life option that is gaining social acceptance is the choice of when to die. This means that a competent adult with a severe and incurable condition without prospect for improvement can request assistance in causing their death. This assistance may be from a physician and/or from other intimate individuals who can provide the support to carry out the process necessary to end a life.

In 2014 Brittany Maynard, a 29-year-old Californian, was diagnosed with terminal brain cancer. Rather than let the illness take its dreadful course she moved to Oregon where the "Death with Dignity" law exempts doctors from prosecution if, when following the legal safeguards, they prescribe life-ending drugs to terminally ill patients who request them. She chose the date of her death at a time before she was incapable of taking the medications on her own and when she was certain her remaining days would be filled with pain and suffering. The publicity of her case increased awareness of this option. California subsequently created a legal process for residents of that state to obtain medications for the purpose of ending their life.

As noted, physician-assisted death is legal in 5 U.S. states, and there are proposed laws to legalize this in many other states. These laws require a patient to have a medical condition, certified by two physicians that give them less than six months left to live. The person must be legally competent (i.e. not be mentally ill) to make the decision. They must be a resident of the state and be capable of self-administering the medication that will cause their death.

Oregon, by passing a "Death with Dignity" ballot proposal in 1994, was the first state that established a legal process to allow a physician to prescribe a lethal dose of a medication that a patient must self-administer. In the first 18 years that this has been allowed (the practice was allowed in 1997 since court deliberations delayed the onset of the law), approximately 1000 people have been helped to die through this legal process. It should be noted that when a person invokes the "death with dignity" laws and proceeds through the legal safeguards to take the medications that will cause their death, the law states that this is not to be considered suicide. (While suicide is not illegal, anyone assisting someone to commit suicide is committing a felony.)

Historically, many doctors have quietly eased terminal agonies by increasing pain relief to life-shortening doses. Under the *doctrine of double effect*, as long as the intention was to relieve suffering rather than hasten death, doctors were rarely considered to have committed a criminal or ethical malfeasance. Physician-assisted death is deemed unethical by the British and American Medical Associations, however. "Nor shall any man's entreaty prevail upon me to administer poison to anyone; neither will I counsel any man to do so," runs the Hippocratic Oath, written nearly 2,500 years ago. Recently the California Medical Association has moved towards a more neutral stance where legal safeguards are provided by "Death with Dignity" laws.

Some European nations have laws permitting physician-assisted death for competent citizens of their nations who request it. In the Netherlands, Belgium, and Luxemburg the patient must be certified by a physician to have a condition that causes unbearable suffering without prospect for improvement. The individual requesting the assistance does not have to be certified as having a terminal condition. Patients do not need to self-administer the lethal medications in these countries, as physicians may give the medications by injection.

Switzerland has the most lenient laws. It has been legal there to assist people in dying since 1942, and the individuals do not have to be Swiss citizens. The law states that assisted death is punishable only when it is done for "selfish" reasons. There are assisted dying clinics specializing in providing the services. A large clinic, *Dignitas*, has developed a reputation for "suicide tourism", since they accept foreigners. More than 1,700 people from more than 40 different countries have traveled to Switzerland and ended their lives there since 1998.

Anyone considering planning their death should have counseling, palliative care, and hospice services readily available. The fears that having legally approved structures for planning a death would undermine the development of end-of-life support services have not been realized. In fact, since Oregon and Washington have passed their "Death with Dignity" laws, there has been a substantial increase in hospice and palliative care services. Care at the end of life has improved for all people, including those who choose to control their death under the laws, and those who do not.

Travel to another state or country in order to have legally approved assistance for a patient controlled death may not be possible or may be impractical and difficult. Brittany Maynard, for example, had to move to Oregon and live there for 6 months in order to establish residency before she could invoke the "Death with Dignity" law. The inability to travel may force a person to take their life early if they have to do it themselves, without medical assistance. This is one of the reasons that laws have been passed. They allow people to delay their deaths knowing they will have the legal structure and support to make a decision later. However, other options do exist for adults, competent to make their own decisions, who have an irremediable and grievous condition.

Voluntarily Stopping Eating and Drinking (VSED)

Stopping all nutritional and fluid intakes—complete fasting—will cause death, usually within one to three weeks depending on an individual's underlying condition. It is legal to cause your own death by so doing. Dehydration is the ultimate cause of death. This method of accelerating dying has been recognized and accepted for a long time. There are many well-publicized reports of individuals with terminal conditions and non-mortal conditions that will lead to a reduced quality of life, who have chosen to hasten their deaths by VSED. People with early dementia have made this choice before they lost the competence to do so, and there are several publicized cases (described in the Journal of the American Medical Association and the New York Times) of elderly people who were "tired of living" who made the decision to stop eating and drinking.

Since VSED is a natural process of dying, people experience a range of symptoms as the dehydration progresses. Most individuals who hasten their death by this approach die peacefully and with dignity according to hospice nurses. An individual who chooses this process will gradually become weaker and have little energy. Some people describe a sense of peace, even euphoria. Others become confused and agitated. Mental alertness recedes and people become very sleepy after the first few days. Most people go in and out of consciousness. The dehydration frequently causes the mouth to dry out and the lips to be parched and cracked, the tongue to swell. There may be nose bleeds. Nausea, vomiting, and abdominal cramps may develop. After several days there may be confusion and agitation. Rarely there are convulsions.

For a VSED death not to be painful and uncomfortable, individuals need medical and other caregivers to support them during the dehydration process. The person may need help because of weakness and light headedness. Medications used to manage pain may need to be continued. Sedatives for anxiety and agitation may be needed, as well as personal help with local discomforts such as moisture for the lips and mouth. 24-hour support will be necessary. Supporters must understand how the fast may progress, and not provide any fluids for this to proceed without actually prolonging the patient's discomfort.

In conclusion, when a person considers a patient controlled death, talking with their family and care providers is important. They need to be aware of her end-of-life wishes, values, and concerns. She can describe to them her suffering and fears about further deterioration of her quality of life. Hospice will usually support these conversations. A consultation with a mental health provider addressing depression and decision making capacity is frequently recommended.

There are organizations that can provide information and consultation about a patient controlled death. **Compassion & Choices** offers such help. They are well experienced and recognized for their support of end-of-life choices, and have built a reputation for their work in this area. They offer and *End of Life Consultation* program. Their U.S. phone number is 800-247-7421 and their web site is www. compassionandchoices.org.

Chapter 9
Advance Directives

This chapter discusses Advance Directives for Health Care. *Advance Directives for Health Care are written documents that express your wishes and instructions to be followed when you are unable to make or state your decisions.* The components of this legal document can include:
- A living will
- A durable power of attorney for health care
- A "do not resuscitate" order (DNR)

Advance directives for health care are an attempt to extend the exercise of your autonomy over medical decision making beyond your span of competence. You may become unable, either temporarily or permanently to participate in making medical decisions. This may happen as a result of an injury, a disease process, or surgery. You may be conscious but unable to communicate, as sometimes happens after a stroke. You may lose the ability to think properly due to dementia. You may be in a coma or may be temporarily unconscious due to a disease like inflammation or infection of the brain (encephalitis) or surgery. The law of every U.S. state provides for advance directives for health care; and the federal law, the Patient Self-Determination Act of 1990, mandates that healthcare facilities of all types advise their clients of their rights and options under these state laws.

The goal of laws supporting advance directives is to provide clarity and a legal structure so that individuals can inform their health care providers of their values and preferences and to keep medical decision making issues out of the courts. The Karen Ann Quinlan case in 1976 and the Nancy Cruzan case in 1988-1990 provided the impetus to develop legal tools so that individuals could make health care decisions when they are capable that would take effect if they became non-competent. These famous cases and others since then have shown that end-of-life decisions can cause much controversy and strife in families. Advance directives offer a way to keep these decisions from causing unnecessary distress in situations which are inherently challenging emotionally.

Your Legal Rights

Case law from the courts, as well as statutory law from legislation, has established that people have a number of rights.

- You can refuse any unwanted treatment, even if this refusal may lead to death. This includes treatments that have not yet been initiated, as well as treatments that are under way that you want to have stopped. Nutrition and hydration support, such as intravenous infusions and tube feedings, are considered treatments and can be stopped. A pacemaker can be turned off.
- You can refuse to have cardiopulmonary resuscitation (CPR).
- You can have medications for pain and suffering, even if death may be the unintended result.
- You can expect your advance directives to be followed. Incompetent patients have the same rights as competent patients that their expressed wishes be respected.
- You can designate a healthcare advocate, or surrogate, to make decisions if you are not physically or mentally capable of making them.
- Your can expect your surrogate to act on your preferences. Advance directives can be expressed in writing or orally. If the surrogate does not have full information about your preferences, the surrogate should approximate what he thinks you would have wanted based on his understanding of your values and wishes. If your preferences are unclear, the surrogate should make a decision in "your best interests" as he understands them.

Despite the notoriety of the court cases including the more recent Terry Schiavo case, and the efforts by legislatures, courts, administrative agencies, medical associations, spiritual groups, and many other organizations to publicize and promote the benefits and wisdom of advance directives, fewer than one-fifth of all adults in the U.S. have prepared these legal documents. And less than half of severely or terminally ill patients had an advance directive in their medical record. In a study of dialysis patients all of whom are considered to be seriously ill, only 35% had a living will. Even though most people are never incapacitated and do not need to invoke advance directives, it is estimated that 100,000 Americans are currently in a permanent vegetative state and are simply being kept alive. Most of these individuals do not have advance directives. A study which reviewed the circumstances of people who died after the age of 60, found that 42.5% required a decision about their care in the last weeks of life and 70.3% lacked the ability to make decisions. This means that about 30% needed a proxy to make decisions for them.

What Prevents Most People From Preparing Advanced Directives?

Why don't people prepare advance directives even though conventional wisdom recommends them? Many explanations are given: they do not know enough about them, they think they are hard to execute, or they are hesitant to broach the subject with their families or their doctors. In a recent study, 91% of armed forces veterans doubted that advance directives would change the treatment they would receive. Others feel they are only for the elderly, the sick, or the infirm. Many people prefer to leave these decisions to their family and physician. In two large studies called the SUPPORT study and the HELP study, involving more than 10,000 patients, only 20-30% of patients would want their own preferences followed, preferring instead to have others make the choices. The topics of being incapacitated or near death elicit unpleasant feelings including fear and anxiety which people prefer to avoid.

Reverend Carney, a Methodist minister, had many times in his career been involved in helping people talk about end-of-life issues. He had led study groups on grief and loss. Yet even after he was living in a retirement community where he had developed a program to help residents of his community with end-of-life issues, he had not talked with his family about his feelings around the end of his own life. When his daughter started to ask him what his preferences and feelings were on this, he started to cry. He said he would just leave it to his children to decide. After being reminded of his experiences in his work of how families can be painfully divided when the advance preparation is not carefully considered, he finally chose to develop his own advance directives. In spite of feeling overwhelmed by his emotions at the start of the process, he was greatly relieved once he had completed his advance directives.

Medicare and Medicaid now pay for a discussion of Advance Care Planning with a primary care physician. When this clause was being discussed during the consideration of the Affordable Care Act, some politicians (Sarah Palin was one) said that this proposal added up to being a "death panel" where the fates of older and disabled individuals would be decided upon. This became a "sound bite".

Sound bites are an attempt to spin information towards a particular bias. This, in decision making parlance, is a type of "heuristic" or short cut that can avoid critical and careful consideration of all the facts. Academics call this particular shortcut the **"availability bias"** (chapter 3). The availability bias is commonly used by politicians, advertisers, and others.

Vivid memories and vivid stories, repeated short bits of information, clever ways of putting words together, even jingles, especially when repeated a number of times, such as in an advertising campaign or a political campaign, are **available**. Information that is frequently in the news is available. This leads to an overestimation of the accuracy of the information and of the impact of this news on our lives.

One of the reasons that Palin's sound bite calling advance care planning a form of a "death panel" gained traction is that discussions of advance care planning frequently take place only at a time when we are entering the hospital or are diagnosed with a serious illness. So then, the suspicions that these discussions are meant to limit our care, to convince us to forgo care and not have needed interventions to keep us alive can easily arise.

Another important reason that talking about "death panels" raised fears is that we have tended to medicalize the dying process. We try to deny death rather than accept that death is really a part of the circle of life. By medicalizing death we attempt to see it as an aberration that needs to be treated and intervened with in an attempt to postpone it. We worry that people will give up too soon. So there is a greater use of medical treatments, intensive care units, life-sustaining devices, and other interventions, even when the probability of success is minimal and the chance of unacceptable outcomes is increased. This is also due to the limited ability to predict the time of the actual death. A lack of feeling certain that it will really happen is common in western cultures. This results in a societal phenomenon of attempting to deny death, and a resistance to talking about it.

But we really cannot escape death! We can escape discomfort and loss of dignity, however.

Sound bites work! They become "available" information. In this case, the use of "death panels" was used to create suspicion and fear, and to discredit the health care reform proposal. Rather than having others decide the fate of individuals, discussions about advanced care planning are just the opposite. I prefer to think of advance care planning as an attempt to extend the right of individuals to make their own choices over the health care they want; an attempt to prevent the theft of your autonomy.

The Living Will

A **living will** is a written statement in which you inform healthcare providers and family members what type of medical care you wish to receive should you become unable to make decisions, and an opportunity to state your wishes about your continued care. In this document, you consider different possible scenarios and state what medical care you want in each of these. This is a daunting task. It is really a guessing game for anyone to consider and understand unknown or unanticipated maladies and unpredictable treatments and diagnostic approaches, be they in a medical field or not. We have difficulty in gathering and understanding information on current situations, so it seems even harder to do this for future, unknown conditions.

In addition, we must try to predict our future preferences and feelings (chapter 3). Studies have shown that within 2 years, one-third of people changed their preferences for life-sustaining treatments. The desire for life-sustaining treatments declined significantly upon being hospitalized, then returned to close to its original level 3 to 6 months after being hospitalized. Interest in life-sustaining treatments shifts over time and situations. People are unable to predict future tastes and feelings about simple and familiar matters such as foods, fashion, or entertainment preferences, so it is unlikely they can predict their preferences about unfamiliar situations that may take place in the future.

Many living wills describe in general terms what the person wishes. A group of patients who had written living wills were asked what their will stated, and the typical answer was: "It says I don't want to be a vegetable." Such general goals are difficult to apply to specific situations. A living will requires clarity and specificity in stating the instructions, but most people know too little about the possible situations they may be in, and the possible choices that will be available. Drafting instructions is thus very difficult.

Drafting a living will, therefore, presents difficulties that compromise its future utility to be a useful legal instrument. However, it can be a useful tool to aid in a discussion of our preferences and values. Particular situations can be imagined, such as being terminally ill with cancer, or being in a coma with a high likelihood of significant mental impairment if you survive, or being in a coma with a very little chance of surviving. If you were to be in such a situation, how would you want to be treated? Would you want antibiotics to treat pneumonia? Would you want intravenous feedings? Would you want pain medication? These discussions, particularly if taking place with the person who will act as your surrogate decision maker, can help both of you to understand your current feelings. Talking about these situations may require someone with medical knowledge to act as a facilitator. To keep your preferences current, these discussions need to be repeated periodically.

Durable Power of Attorney for Health Care

A **durable power of attorney for health care** is a document in which you give another person the power to make decisions regarding medical treatment and related personal matters for you if you are not able to do so for yourself. The living will describes **what** you would want to be done and the durable power of attorney designates **who** you would want to see that it is done. This authority delegated to your "patient-advocate" (another term for the surrogate) is triggered at the onset of your inability to state your instructions. This is a powerful document. The person making decisions for you must understand your values and preferences, and must be willing to represent them to the medical providers. You must trust this person to be able to do this.

The patient-advocate can make decisions regarding your need to have nursing care. She can decide to continue or withdraw life-sustaining treatment, such as a ventilator. She can decide to continue or withdraw food and water. She may decide to proceed or discontinue treatments and interventions for you.

The patient-advocate should promote health care decisions as they understand your preferences to be. These may have been expressed in writing, either in a *living will* or in the *durable power of attorney for health care* document, or may have been expressed orally. Recent legal decisions have stated that "clear and convincing evidence" can be provided by witnesses to your oral statements, and that these are legally binding and should be carried out. If there is no information about what your preferences are in a given situation, then the advocate should use her best judgment to determine what you would have wanted. This advocate can make a decision in what she understands to be your best interests. The best way to assure that your preferences are put into effect if the need arises is to **choose an advocate who shares your views and values**. It is also a good idea to discuss this periodically. Of course, the advocate has to agree to serve in this role.

The choice of a **patient-advocate also must be someone who is likely to be available** when the need arises. One study found that in 30 of 39 cases in which patients needed decisions to be made by a surrogate and had a durable power of attorney document in place, the available surrogate decision maker in these cases was not the person named in the power of attorney document. The person named in the document was either not available, or was overwhelmed and was unable to advocate effectively for the patient.

Jane, a vigorous woman in her mid 70's had signed advance directives and placed them in her medical record. She also gave copies to her three children. She had made clear statements that she did not want efforts to sustain her life if it was likely that survival of any serious illness would result in brain damage that would cause her to be dependent on others. In particular, she did not want to end up with difficulties in her thinking and memory. Her advance directives said her children were to have the decision making power. When she suddenly developed an infection of her brain (meningoencephalitis), she became comatose and was hospitalized. A few days after the disease became manifest, when the treatment was not having the desired effects and she was still in a coma, the doctors told her children that she was highly likely to have significant brain damage if she survived. There was a choice at that time to stop her treatments which would probably lead to her death.

Her oldest son was adamant that her living will preferences were not yet to be invoked because she was not moribund and it was not completely clear what the resultant brain damage would be. He felt that she was not hopelessly ill. There was strong disagreement between the siblings. This meant that the medical treatment would continue until the differences among them were resolved. No resolution occurred and three weeks later, Jane came out of her coma and survived her disease. But she had lost much of her memory, could speak but not clearly, and was unable to care for herself. She has been placed in a nursing home. The children still disagree and have strong feelings about the assessment of the outcome. The eldest feels he was right, that she still may improve. The others feel that their mother's clearly expressed wishes were violated and she is living with the impaired abilities that she wanted to avoid.

It is possible that a durable power of attorney for health care that specifically named who the advocate would have been may have avoided this family disagreement. These difficult situations, however, can sometimes not be resolved, even with advance planning and open discussions. It is worth making efforts to avoid adding family disagreements and divisions to these painful and complex problems. Yet discussions with primary care providers, within families, and in spiritual communities about advance directives and planning are rare. People too often just want to avoid thinking about this. You should select as a patient-advocate one person for this role only, in order to avoid dividing the responsibility between several people. An alternate choice, should your first-named advocate be unavailable, should also be named in the document. This can help avoid the sort of conflict, and confusion, experienced by Jane's children.

Do Not Resuscitate Order

The **do not resuscitate order (DNR)** can be important when someone is approaching the end of life. It refers to resuscitation when heart or lung function ceases (a cardio-pulmonary arrest). It does not impede efforts to "resuscitate" with fluids when someone is dehydrated or with a blood transfusion if someone is severely depleted of blood. If you do not want efforts to do cardio-pulmonary resuscitation (CPR) in the event your heart and lung stop functioning, this order is essential. Healthcare providers feel obligated to resuscitate unless they are certain that a decision not to proceed with efforts to restore heart and lung activity has been documented. If an ambulance or emergency unit is called, personnel will feel obligated to make efforts to resuscitate without this document being available to them.

CPR is a physical procedure that can be quite traumatic. The chances of success of this procedure depend on the underlying condition of the person having the arrest. Survival to discharge from a hospital after a CPR procedure for those who have underlying conditions such as heart failure, cancer, neurological afflictions, or advanced age alone (over 75 years old) is very small: from 1-3%. If a person survives to discharge, frequently there are permanent cognitive or physical consequences from the arrest and procedure that can be severe and incapacitating. Following a CPR procedure, because it is traumatic and can cause rib fractures and other injuries, there can be significant pain if the person survives for a period of time after the procedure.

The laws regarding DNR vary from state to state. A physician's signature is almost always required for documents that refer to either in-hospital or out-of-hospital CPR. (Some states have laws that require separate DNR orders if the cardio-pulmonary arrest occurs while a person is hospitalized rather than in the community.) If a person wishes to avoid these aggressive and sometimes traumatic efforts to revive them, then DNR document must be accessible immediately. Bracelets are available stating you do not want CPR (and that you have prepared documents stating this) that is worn on the arm or leg and make that information immediately available. Emergency crews will still provide palliative support such as oxygen and pain relief even if DNR orders are followed. Many retirement communities and assisted-living or nursing home institutions have mechanisms for making these orders accessible.

What if You Don't Sign or Provide an Advance Directive?

Someone has to make decisions when an ill person cannot. Without directives in the person's medical record or hospital files, and without the appointment of a surrogate decision maker through a durable power of attorney, your doctors, hospital staff and loved ones will do the best they can. For your spouse, child, or life-long friend, this might mean struggling with what they think you would want. To the medical staff, it means letting their training and professional experience guide them. Unfortunately, in a world of good intentions, that training has traditionally led health care professionals to do all they can to keep a person alive. All too often, well-meaning health professionals make medical decisions for a patient who is not competent to do this for himself, based on their own personal and religious beliefs rather than on their knowledge and understanding of what the patient would have wanted.

Recent laws are making it easier for these professionals to find the best ways to make you comfortable. However, the ways that they interpret the laws may not be what you want. Sometimes, especially when a catastrophic condition persists for a long time, a conservator (or guardian) may be appointed by a court to make these decisions if a surrogate decision maker cannot be identified. A request for designation of a conservator must be made to a court if your family cannot be located. The conservator, which might be a public agency, would then make decisions about health care.

We can never really know how much longer we have left to live. Having conversations about your end of life choices should not wait. Discussing your advance directives and planning for future care has benefits. Several studies have shown that people who discussed this with their families and doctors had less fear and anxiety about their future healthcare needs. They were more confident that their wishes would be considered if they were incapacitated, and families had a greater agreement about end-of-life-care issues. People who had conversations about their preferences with their doctors were more likely to die in peace and in some control over their situation. They suffered less pain and were more likely to die at home. They had better interactions with their family members and spared them anguish. Plus after their death, close family members were less likely to suffer from depression.

Once advance directives are prepared, it is valuable to place these documents in several places. It is important to give copies to your doctors. In one study 70% of the doctors of patients who had prepared advance directives were unaware of their existence. A copy should be readily available to take to a hospital or nursing home. Advance directives assisted in making end-of-life decisions in less than half the cases for patients who *had* prepared these directives because these were not readily available. The advocate named in the durable power of attorney for health care also should have a copy.

Conclusions

Advance Directives can inform the persons who care for you what your wishes are when you are not able to articulate them. The decision which is most important in ensuring that your wishes are carried out is the choice of your patient-advocate or surrogate decision maker. A durable power of attorney is the instrument in which to name this person. Copies of these advance directives should be readily available to those who will be caring for you and making decisions for you. Your patient-advocate should be a person who is likely to be available should you become incapacitated. Your surrogate should be clear as to what your desires are, and should be willing to invoke them should the situation arise. A person who has different values and beliefs than yours may be unable to make decisions on your behalf that would violate their values, so choose carefully and discuss them beforehand.

Section 4

Planning and Clarifying

Gathering medical information that is reliable and up to date is no easy task. If you are well informed, however, you can be a more competent participant in making decisions regarding your health care. A cornerstone of *informed choice* depends on patients (or their surrogate decision makers if the patient is not capable) having an understanding of their medical situation and the possible impact the different options for managing their condition will have on both their quality of life and life expectancy. This section provides tools and ideas to use in gathering reliable information.

Also, in this section, we'll consider particular situations that require decision making. You'll learn what it means to agree to be a participant in a research trial if that is an option is offered to you. We'll also explore how to choose a health care provider when seeking specialty care or second opinions, which may be an important decision in obtaining high-quality health care.

Chapter 10

Gathering Information

You will need to **gather reliable information** in order to make informed medical decisions. There are many sources of medical information you can choose from including:
- The world wide web or internet
- Physicians and specialists, including the option of obtaining second opinions
- Medical and professional journals
- Medical textbooks

The general news media
Books on medical information for the general public

The Internet

In a recent search for "depression" via that source of medical expertise which has become ubiquitous, the search engine Google, one of the web sites listed near the top identified the cause of depression as sin! Other sites offered a variety of treatments for depression, many without evidence of efficacy. An additional 237,000,000 hits in that search yielded a dizzying array of added information. The **World Wide Web (WWW)** is a huge and at times overwhelming source of information. The search engines, such as Google and Yahoo, will list close to a billion web sites, if you search for health information using various headings like "health" or "health care" (defined as the prevention, treatment, and management of illness and the preservation of mental and physical well-being through the services offered by the medical and allied health professions). The search engines have become increasingly sophisticated and capable of responding to detailed requests so that a particular article or author can be singled out in a search. We can now focus the searches with greater precision for the information we may be seeking.

As noted, search engines provide lists of many web sites in response to information we place in the search bar. It is known that the first few listed are most frequently the ones viewed by the searcher. So if you want your site viewed as much as possible, it is to your advantage to have it listed near the top. There are strategies that cause a site to be listed higher during searches that web designers can use. Service providers offering to improve your ranking exist. Clearly, the placement on the list has no correlation with the quality or reliability of the information offered on a web site.

A Harvard information technology group and others who have studied medical web sites estimate that *95% or more of health care information on the net is either simply not trustworthy or outright bogus.* Information on these sites is considered incomplete or biased because they are based on belief rather than on science. They may be selling a product or a service such as some of the treatments offered for depression, which makes them interested in having readers believe their material. Even with this large number of unreliable or corrupt sites, it still means that many thousands of web pages do offer reliable information on health issues. However, it is difficult for most people to distinguish good and reliable information from that which is incomplete or incorrect.

Reliable Web Sites

There are excellent web sites which can help you obtain both general information and specialized material. High-quality web sites which are well maintained so that the information is up to date, reviewed regularly by acknowledged experts, and complete, usually originate from sources we can trust. Our confidence in the source is based on advice from people we respect, from past experiences, and from reputation. For example, the U.S., United Kingdom, Canadian, and

Australian governments run medical information sites in English that are well maintained, up to date, and contain reliable information. They do not accept advertising. They do not have a profit incentive. Academic institutions such as universities and many highly regarded health care organizations also host reliable and well-maintained sites.

The following sites I have found useful and reliable for many different types of health care information and information on research in their areas of interest.

- The **National Library of Medicine** offers a large variety of information and resources on a broad range of medical subjects through http://www.nlm.nih.gov/medlineplus/.
- Healthfinder.gov, which provides current news, a health library, and much more, (also available in Spanish) is a **U.S. government** site that has current information on many areas of medical care.
- General health information is available from the **Mayo Clinic** at http://www.mayoclinic.org/.
- **Stanford University** offers a site to search the medical literature for articles through highwire.stanford.edu/lists/freeart.dtl.
- The **Cochrane Collaboration** is an international library dedicated to making up-to-date, evidence-based information about the effects of healthcare readily available worldwide at www.cochrane.org/.
- **The National Institute of Mental Health** provides information on mental disorders at www.nimh.nih.gov/.
- https://www.mskcc.org/cancer-care/treatments/symptom-management/integrative-medicine/herbs from the **Memorial Sloan-Kettering Cancer Center** provides evidence-based information on herbs and botanicals as alternative sources of medical treatments.
- Information on **alternative and complementary medicine**, including current research trials and other news, is available at from the National Institute of Health at https://nccih.nih.gov/from their National Center for Complimentary and Integrative Health.
- **The Centers for Disease Control and Prevention** provides travel health information as well as a wide variety of other information at http://www.cdc.gov/travel.

- **Immunization Action Coalition** provides immunization and vaccination information for all age groups at http://www. immunize.org/.
- You can search for current **clinical research studies** on many different conditions in the U.S at www.clinicaltrials.gov.
- **The American Heart Association** is a resource for cardiovascular disease; information at www.heart.org/HEARTORG/.
- **The National Cancer Institute** focuses on cancer types, treatments and clinical trials at www.cancer.gov.
- A virtual atlas of the human body can be found at http://www. ikonet.com/en/health/virtual-human-body/virtualhumanbody.php.
- A reliable web site sponsored by **Harvard University** information is http://www.health.harvard.edu/.
- The National Health Service from the UK has developed a web site to provide independent expert commentaries on topical medical matters reported in the international news media at http://www. nhs.uk/news/Pages/NewsIndex.aspx/.
- National Institute for Health and Care Excellence (NICE) from the UK provides evidence-based guidance on many medical conditions at nice.org.uk.

Some web sites have offered good information at one point, yet have become commercialized and do not keep their web sites up to date due to financial constraints. These are mostly web sites that had hoped to make money by having paid advertisements. The site *drkoop.com* was one of the first major online sources of health information. Initially founded by Dr. C. Everett Koop in 1998 after he was Surgeon General of the U.S., and supported by other investors, it earned a reputation for being innovative and reliable. It was ranked the number 1 health information web site in 1999 and had many daily users. Later they had financial problems which resulted in staff cuts, and their information became dated and the site was not well maintained. A critical review of the site content at that time revealed that many of the private care listings, medicinal recommendations, and medical trial referrals were in fact paid advertisements! It shut down its operations in 2001.

The power of the internet to provide vast amounts of information easily has led to some unanticipated consequences. One newly termed condition is being called "**cyberchondria**". A study done by Microsoft revealed that self-diagnosis based on health information obtained through a web search can lead the searcher to conclude that he is suffering from the worst possible disease that has similar symptoms to those he is experiencing. **Cyberchondria** refers to this practice of leaping to dire conclusions while researching health matters online. This can lead to significant anxiety since the searcher now feels certain that he is seriously ill. If he has a headache, he may believe he has a brain tumor, since headaches are cited as one of the symptoms of brain tumors, even though the likelihood of this is infinitesimally small. It is much more likely that he is suffering from the symptoms of caffeine withdrawal (a common cause of a headache), or a tension headache.

The examination of search records by the Microsoft researchers indicated that searching for information related to particular symptoms often lead quickly to anxiety. Since web searches only match a term or word with sites that contain that word or term, the results do not offer any perspective on the likelihood that the matched site will suggest the probable cause of the symptom in question. Web searches may offer possible causes, but not the likelihood that the symptoms you are experiencing and searching for are caused by any particular medical condition or disease.

Second Opinions

Obtaining a **second opinion** is an important means of seeking more information. Larry was in his late 50's and had painful arthritis in his right hip. He had to stop playing tennis due to the pain. He consulted an arthritis specialist who felt that hip replacement would offer the only way to be pain-free when he walked. He was referred to an orthopedic surgeon who agreed with the recommendation. But he told Larry that with the current and commonly used artificial hips, he would not be able to play tennis or participate in similar sports in the future because of the risk of dislocating the new joint. He asked for a second opinion with an orthopedic surgeon at a medical school in a nearby city who his original specialist had also recommended. This second orthopedic surgeon told him his department was starting to use a new "resurfacing" procedure for hip replacements which created a larger and more stable joint. While this procedure was new for orthopedists in the U.S. and considered investigational (since the FDA had not yet approved the new hip prosthesis device), it had been used in England for more than 10 years. After doing research on this procedure, Larry chose to proceed with the resurfacing. He realized that there is some risk in having a new technical procedure performed, where experience is limited. But he has had an excellent result and is playing doubles tennis again. One significant drawback was that since it was considered investigational and not FDA-approved, his insurance company refused to cover the costs and he had to pay nearly $25,000 to have this done.

You can obtain an alternative point of view when you consult a doctor from a different medical specialty, and this perspective frequently provides information that can help you make a wise medical decision. Every specialist has a "bias" that is based on their experience, training, and interests. They must preferentially concentrate on the literature and new information from their specialty groups. Particularly, when you are facing a major decision, a second opinion can provide information that may assist in either confirming the diagnosis or in choosing the best treatment option. You may be given conflicting opinions by the different specialists. In which case, you may have to decide what choice is best for you. This may require you to get additional information or advice from a source you trust. It may even be necessary to get an opinion from another specialist! There are controversies in medicine that are difficult to resolve.

John, a 54-year-old financial expert, developed severe and persistent back pain. After 6 weeks, the pain was continuing to cause him to restrict his activities and made it difficult to sleep through the night. He consulted a spine surgeon who specialized in back pain. The MRI (magnetic resonance image) the surgeon ordered revealed a herniated disc in the region of his pain, and he recommended surgery to remove the disc. His personal doctor felt he should have a second opinion and referred him to a specialist in physical medicine. This physiatrist's opinion, after a careful examination, was that a conservative approach was appropriate. This meant staying as active as possible, taking mild pain medication, and having a physical therapy program. This would provide safe treatment for the problem, and he would probably avoid surgery. John followed this advice and was back to his normal activity without pain in 12 weeks. Doctors recommend what they know and have experience with. Surgeons tend to recommend surgery. A medical specialist is less likely to do so. Back pain is a common malady, causing much pain and disability and many visits to doctors. There are differing opinions as to the treatment which is the safest or that will yield the quickest benefits. John successfully avoided surgery by seeking a second opinion from an alternative point of reference.

Specialists and specialty clinics in medical centers frequently have teams who work under the supervision of specialist doctors. These teams, including nurse practitioners, physician assistants, and nurses who are trained in the specialty, and play different roles in evaluating and in educating patients about their options and treatments for the various ailments they specialize in. They can provide invaluable information about the medical conditions and can take the time to discuss information and be sure you understand their explanations. Frequently, printed materials are available from them. They can provide ways for you to get back in touch with their clinics (such as by email or telephone), making it possible to ask questions as they arise, even after you are home.

Requesting a second opinion may feel difficult for you. You may feel embarrassed or afraid to ask for a second opinion for fear it will weaken your relationship with your doctor or create ill feelings. You may feel that you are expressing a lack of confidence in the first opinion. You may fear that doctors may be hurt or offended by your request. Health insurance companies and other sources of medical payments may consider second opinions to be an unnecessary waste of money and resources, though usually, they are glad that you are researching your options and not jumping to conclusions about treatments that may have unnecessary risks and costs. Research suggests that concern about requesting second opinions is unwarranted. When important decisions, such as the diagnosis and treatment of cancer or the need for major surgery are reassessed, a substantial number of differences between the original decision from the first consultant and the second opinion are found. Many initial decisions are reversed. Patient outcomes, including satisfaction with care, tend to improve and cost of care does not increase. There may be savings to the system by avoiding unnecessary procedures. I feel second opinions can be of great importance and are worth the investment of time and money.

Many individuals have concerns about how to inform their physicians that they have chosen a different option than the original recommendation they were offered. Being clear about your preferences and choices should not harm these relationships. Many physicians are pleased to receive requests for second opinions. Their own uncertainties can be eased by having another physician express a view. They can also have an opportunity to obtain information and learn from the second consultant. The primary care physician may offer to consult with another specialist on his own, or may provide you with the names of doctors from whom to seek a second opinion. Many insurance companies are now paying for these services, as they realize that it improves outcomes and tends to save money. Medicare will pay 80% of the cost. As a matter of fact, if the second opinion doesn't agree with the first, Medicare will pay 80% of the cost of a third opinion. Some insurance programs actually require a second opinion prior to approving a major and costly intervention.

Current Medical Textbooks and Medical Journals

Current medical textbooks and medical journals can yield good information. Since medical information is expanding rapidly, it is important to seek recent publications and editions. Medical texts exist that are particular to different specialties. They are usually updated periodically by issuing new editions. You can check their copyright dates to see how recent the text you are referring too has been updated.

Well known journals in English include **The New England Journal of Medicine, Journal of the American Medical Association,** and **the Lancet**, as well as the journals of many medical specialty societies. These journals are thorough and rigorous in their choices of medical articles; so that we can be confident they are reporting on investigations of high quality and are really adding value and knowledge to the vast medical information available. They set standards of objectivity, reproducibility, methodology, and statistical computations to assure that each article offers reliable and confirmable information. The web sites of these journals allow you to search for journal articles by subjects or titles. They provide sources you can trust. (This does not mean they are infallible in the choices of their articles. In chapter 1 I discuss an article from **the Lancet** that was later retracted. **The Lancet** also published an editorial expressing regret for their error.)

The methods of investigation for studies published in reliable journals set strict boundaries for the investigation, often limiting the conclusions that can be made. For example, a study of middle-aged men with coronary artery disease found that using statin medications to markedly lower cholesterol levels lowers the risk of a subsequent heart attack. This true scientific conclusion cannot be said to apply to men who do not have proven coronary artery disease, nor to women, since these groups were not studied in this clinical study. Yet newspaper reports of this study have generalized the results to say "aggressive lowering of cholesterol is the best way to prevent a heart attack," since such generalized statements gather more attention. (There have been other studies of the impact of statins on subjects with different boundary conditions such as past medical conditions and genders that have provided scientific information about these groups.)

Reading from medical texts and medical journals can prove challenging, though. They use technical language, and it can take years to become familiar with "medicalese" and the formats of these resources (see Supplementary Material on medical terminology). You may find it necessary to have someone translate the information from medical journals and texts into a language you can understand and to make certain it can apply to your situation, before it can be useful in reaching a medical decision. This translator can be your personal physician, a friend with a background in the health professions, or a health care advocate.

Newspapers and Television News

An astounding article in a popular medical column in a local newspaper stated that cherry juice was an effective and inexpensive treatment for arthritis and gout with no side effects. A study had found several antioxidants in tart cherries which appeared to have an inhibiting effect on some of the enzymes associated with gout and arthritis, when they were examined in a test tube. These enzymes are produced by humans and can increase chemical substances that are present in the damaged joints of arthritis sufferers. But research in humans has not yet been done to determine whether cherries will actually be able to inhibit these enzymes in humans. So although it works in a test tube, there is no evidence at all that cherries can relieve actual arthritis symptoms. Yet this column sounded authoritative and reasonable. It did not include any disclaimers or reservations. Cherry producers were probably pleased to see this treatment suggestion in the popular press!

Information from the **news media** on health issues is widely available. Articles on health care are among the most frequently read subjects appearing in newspapers. The **general news media** provides substantial coverage of scientific meetings and publications. Too often, however, the media focus is on getting attention for their message rather than getting their message right. The mass-media reports on health are as reliable as the reports on all other subjects. Readers (that is, buyer) beware!

News reports often bring new medical information to the public before their validity and importance has been established in the scientific community. They report on findings discussed in a meeting before they have been verified and published in the medical literature. They are looking for a "scoop". The studies on which they are basing their newspaper stories may not yet have been reviewed by other researchers. They may contradict earlier reports on the same subject, and they may write articles based on small or weakly designed studies, or on studies looking at animals and not humans. Because the findings the news media choose to report on may be spectacular and bring more attention from readers, they are considered "newsworthy". Yet many reports in the mass news media are never verified (or shown they can be reproduced which is necessary for scientific verification) or ever published in scientific publications! Prominent medical journal editors have expressed concern that newspapers' reporting of health issues attributes too much certainty to research findings, prematurely claim early findings to be breakthroughs, and are often alarmist, incomplete, or simply wrong.

However, there are good articles in the *Health* sections of newspapers. They can give a perspective on some of the controversies and uncertainties in medicine. These helpful articles seldom are based on one scientific report or study. Instead, they look at a body of information based on a number of published reports. They typically provide diverse opinions on a topic from different points of view, by interviewing different specialists and researchers and balancing their responses. Gina Kolata, who has been reporting on health issues for the *New York Times* for a number of years, is an example of such a writer. Her articles provide a broad perspective on controversies in medicine without over-interpreting or reaching premature conclusions. Look for this sort of balanced journalism as you educate yourself about health topics related to your personal concerns.

Books on Medical Subjects Written for the Public

Books on medical subjects written for the general public are available on virtually any topic. The information is often presented from a particular point of view or based on one person's experience. Such books become dated very quickly. Medical knowledge and medical science is changing and expanding quickly. A few years ago, books gave advice for menopausal women to take hormone replacements. Now it is felt that these hormone replacements offer risks that generally exceed the benefits. Vitamin E was touted as being beneficial. Now the evidence from several well-designed studies is convincing that there are potential harms and little benefit in taking it. Regularly updated information resources, such as internet websites that are well maintained and medical journals, can report new information as it is gathered, but books tend to stay in libraries and home collections for many years. In general, books are not a reliable source of information when you are trying to make a medical decision about a particular problem.

Pseudoscience

There are many books, magazine articles, and a number of internet sites that offer information regarded by many as **pseudoscience**. Pseudoscience is any body of alleged knowledge, methodology, belief, or practice that is presented as scientific, but fails to meet the norms for scientific research or is unsupported by adequate scientific research to justify its claims. It may be supported by personal anecdotes or apparent logic, but not with evidence. Promoters of pseudoscience generally fail to make the documentation of data and methodology available for close and repeated scrutiny by other scientists and researchers. Nor do they make available any other relevant information used to arrive at particular results. Thus it can't be determined if the claims are verifiable and reproducible, which are essential aspects of the scientific method. There is no scientific validity to claims which cannot be verified and reproduced.

An example of a form of pseudoscience which is now discredited is phrenology. It was popular in the 1800s. Phrenology claims to be able to determine character, personality traits, intelligence, and criminality on the basis of the shape of the head (reading "bumps"). The idea was that our traits were based on different aspects of our mind. Different parts of our organ of mind, the brain, would be more prominent depending on the trait or character being prominently expressed in that person. That characteristic would be reflected by the overlying skull being prominent in that spot. This "science" was used in anthropology and ethnology. Among others, it justified racist ideas by qualifying as inferior some people who had characteristics in the shape of their heads based on race that was believed to reveal inferiority. This was a very popular pseudoscience which was widely reported and widely embraced, in spite of the lack of evidence to support it.

Some of the characteristics that help identify pseudoscience include the use of vague, exaggerated, or untestable claims, and the assertion of scientific claims that are imprecise and that lack specific measurements as a basis. Many proponents of pseudoscience use grandiose or highly technical jargon in an effort to provide their disciplines with the superficial trappings of science, so their language sounds precise and scientific. They may also lack what are considered "boundary conditions". Most well-supported scientific theories possess clear limits under which the predicted phenomena do and do not apply. In contrast, many pseudoscientific phenomena are purported to operate across an exceedingly wide range of conditions. So, if it is good for "whatever ails you" or it sounds too good to be believed, it is probably not based on sound science and should not be accepted.

An example that fits many of the characteristics that define pseudoscience in medicine is illustrated by laetrile, also known as amygdalin. Laetrile is a chemical substance extracted from almond or apricot pits, sometimes referred to as vitamin B 17. It has been promoted as an effective treatment for cancer. The promoters have provided the precise chemical formula and have explained in scientific language how this molecule was effective in treating cancerous tumors in mice as well as anecdotal evidence of effective treatment in humans. Clinics sprang up in Mexico offering this treatment. Yet clinical trials did not reveal any benefit from this treatment and actually caused harm and possibly the premature deaths of some patients. A number of respected groups have stated that there is no sound evidence that laetrile is effective. The American Cancer Society has officially labeled laetrile as quackery.

A number of currently accepted scientific theories were once rejected by mainstream scientists and mathematicians of their time as being pseudoscientific, irrational or obviously false. These include the big bang theory, the theory of continental drift, the theory of black holes, and others. Pseudoscience can become accepted science once the methods used and boundaries applied reveal reproducible information.

Chapter 11

Participation in Clinical Research

Let's consider the possibility of becoming a patient-subject in a research trial. You need to understand what it means to be in a clinical trial. You need to understand what it may offer you in the diagnosis and treatment of your medical conditions as well as what it may cost you to be a participant in a research program. Understanding this can support you in making a wise decision regarding this option for your medical care.

Sometimes doctors offer patients the opportunity to enroll in a clinical research study. The option is even used as a marketing tool at well-known medical centers. For example, the MD Anderson Cancer Center in Texas cites on their website that participation in investigational research trials is "one of the treatment opportunities" they offer to prospective patients. The suggestion is that a patient may have the newest treatments even before they are available to the general public, by participating in a clinical trial.

There is great interest in clinical research. Trials of diagnostic tests and vaccinations and treatments for many different conditions are ongoing around the world. Trials are supported by governments, by private corporations, by academic institutions, and by a variety of foundations. There are websites that can help individuals search by medical condition for potential trials to participate in as patients (See Website table in the Supplementary Materials and Chapter 10). The opportunity to become a patient-subject in an investigational trial deserves careful consideration of the particulars of the trial and your personal medical situation and the more general issues that surround such participation that will be discussed.

Barbara has advanced metastatic breast cancer. There are tumors in her bones, in her skin, and in her liver. She has been treated with surgery and a number of chemotherapy regimens. When her tumors started to grow again while she was taking one group of medications, the treatment was changed to an alternate group of medications. Of course, each regimen, which can damage cancer cells and keep tumors in check, causes harm to healthy cells as well, and can make a patient feel quite sick. But over the past five years, Barbara has been able to survive and stay active, probably because the treatments have slowed the growth of her tumors and reduced the spread of new ones. Her ability to live with her cancer and continue to have a fairly active life is, in part, due to the learning from many research studies that have been done on breast cancer patients. These studies have revealed the risks and benefits of new treatments and determined the best doses of these medications. But Barbara has been told that there are really no good FDA-approved alternatives available for her now that her breast cancer has become resistant to the last group of medications she has received.

If there are no federally (FDA) approved treatments that have been shown to help patients with breast cancer like hers, Barbara wonders if there are research studies that might offer her new treatment possibilities that may have therapeutic benefits. This is a question that many people with chronic and serious conditions ask, particularly if the current treatment available for them is less than adequate. People with problems that have a major impact on their quality of life, and a significant risk of premature death (such as diabetes, chronic lung problems, different forms of deforming arthritis, heart failure, chronic hepatitis, AIDS, blood diseases, as well as with a variety of cancers) wonder if they might get better results with treatments that are still experimental.

Therapeutic Misconception

There is a perception that investigational trials provide the most modern and cutting-edge treatments that are not available in ordinary medical care. New advances from clinical studies are frequently reported in the news media. Major newspapers feature a *Health* section regularly, and it is one of the most popular parts of the newspaper. In these sections, the new successes in medical treatments are written about. Stories are told of individuals with deadly diseases who had failed the standard treatments, but had dramatic improvements with the new treatments which they received by participating in research studies. Their descriptions of a new lease on life after the death sentence had been pronounced have great human interest. Television news tells these stories as well. This leads to the **"therapeutic misconception"** that investigational treatments offer the best means to have improved outcomes for the participants of the research.

Therapeutic misconception exists in the minds of the public as well as of physicians and scientists. It serves as an inducement to recruit patient-subjects by medical practitioners and investigators. Physician-investigators are naturally enthusiastic about their research and communicate this to us. It also gives all practicing physicians something to offer when there are no other effective ways to treat or fix medical conditions. The possibility that better care and more comprehensive care can be obtained by becoming a patient-subject is an incentive to participate in clinical trials for individual patients. Organizers of some trials even pay medical practitioners a "finder's fee" for each subject they recruit for a study.

The fact is that most investigational trials do not result in therapeutic benefit, but the news media rarely report this. Sometimes major toxicities or harm result from the treatments. Sometimes patients die from participating in these trials. There certainly are trials that show substantial benefits, but they are the minority. For example, only 5% of all cancer drugs that enter initial clinical testing trials are eventually found to be safe and effective enough to gain approval by the Food and Drug Administration (FDA). There is a saying in medical science that "research is like going up an alley to discover whether it is a blind alley or not. Most of the time they are blind alleys."

Why do we not hear more about the research that fails to show benefit? It is more exciting and more interesting to read about the new successes! Bottom line: reporting about success sells more newspapers and advertisements! It boosts the stock of the pharmaceutical companies, too!

Publication bias is the tendency for editors to handle positive experimental results (they found something important or good) differently from results that were negative (found that something did *not* happen or that something bad happened) or inconclusive. The bias towards reporting studies that have positive results is furthered because scientists tend to publish the studies that show measurable positive effects more than they report on studies that have no detectable effect, or have negative effects. They are less inclined to report disappointing results. Pharmaceutical companies that support and perform research have been known to submit studies for publications that show therapeutic benefit and to keep the ones with no promise (hence no likelihood of profits) in their file cabinets. This has been referred to as "the file drawer problem", the tendency for negative or inconclusive results to remain hidden and unpublished. This bias has been shown to exist in the mass news media as well as in scientific publications.

Research Methods and Autonomy

Research is vital to increase knowledge in science, and in the long run, the knowledge gained from clinical research benefits all of us. But the orientation of clinical trials is significantly different from that of standard medical care. Research is devoted to answering specific questions. To do this, the methods must be rigorous and repeatable. So research subjects (the patients) are grouped according to the different treatments, and each individual is assigned to their group through a process of random selection. Much of the time even the doctors running the trial do not know which treatment each participant is receiving. This is called a *blind randomized trial* and is considered the most rigorous scientific test. Some participants may receive medications that are placebos (no active ingredients) or receive medications that are available through standard care, while other groups may receive the experimental medications the trial is evaluating in various doses.

For scientific methodology reasons, flexibility in the dosage of any medication, or the use of additional medications, is usually limited. Also, the laboratory procedures such as blood tests, x-rays, and biopsies are done to measure the outcomes of the trial, not individual responses. So these laboratory procedures are part of the trial design, done as a routine for all, and not based on the individual needs of the patients. The risk of these tests and interventions required by the trial's design is not considered for the individual patients, even though, in general, the studies are designed to minimize risks to participants. All studies are subject to scrutiny and oversight by Institutional Review Boards which work hard to assure that ethical and safety considerations guide the study methods.

Once you choose to participate in an investigational trial, you surrender your autonomy. The choices of treatments and procedures are set by the trial protocol and do not consider individual needs or preferences. The principles of beneficence and non-maleficence that govern standard medical care (to maximize benefits and limit harms to each patient) are not the same in clinical investigations. In clinical research, the ethical principles are primarily concerned with promoting the well-being of future patients. The goal is to benefit *future* patients and society. Research done with scientific methods is an important mechanism to gain evidence and knowledge that can be translated into clinical practice in the future.

It should be clear that there are great efforts made to limit the possible risks of harm to which individuals might be exposed as a result of participation in a research trial. Each investigation must be approved by a committee (called an Institutional Review Board or IRB) which carefully reviews the study methods to ensure that each participant is fully informed of the study plans and potentials for harm to them. The IRB also examines the details of the planned trial to minimize risks of adverse effects to the participants, before the study can be initiated. As the trial is run, the IRB periodically reviews the data on the participants to see if undue harm is noticed, and if so may stop the trial.

Investigational treatments may have clinically meaningful benefits. Patient-subjects may experience reduced pain, increased appetite, and more energy. The treatments may promote weight gain, reduce fatigue, or increase the ability to perform daily activities. The investigational treatment may cause a remission of the disease being treated and potentially extend life. Some of these benefits might accrue from research participation itself. For some people, contributing to research and potentially helping future patients may be an important psychological or spiritual benefit. Taking part in a research study may be a way of acting on charitable or generous instincts which are important to you.

These trials require close observation of the effects of any intervention. The support of doctors, nurses, and other staff running the trial for the participants is, therefore, frequently more robust than standard care, which can provide comfort and improvement due to their care and concern. There may be comfort from being part of a team with a purpose, in addition.

At the same time, participation in a research program may involve burdens. There may be multiple visits, long hours at the clinic, unpleasant procedures, and possibly financial costs associated with participation in research studies. (Some trials require participants to pay for transportation and lodging, and participants may also lose time from work.) The risk of death or severe toxic effects from the investigational treatment is also possible.

As Barbara explored her potential participation in a clinical investigation, it became clear that the benefits of enrolling in a clinical trial were for future patients and society at large. It was clear to her that there would be risks and discomforts in her participation. She understood that she would give up some of the flexibility and choices of standard medical care. She also felt fortunate that many patient-subjects had participated in studies that led to the advances in the treatments of breast cancer that she had benefited from. She decided to become a subject in a trial of a new medication to treat breast cancer. She was given pills to take at precise times of the day. But she has no idea whether she is taking the investigational drug, a placebo, or one of the medications she has previously taken and is no longer controlling her cancer. As a participant, Barbara has surrendered her role in making decisions regarding her own treatment once she decided to take part in clinical research. She does know she has the right to withdraw from her participation in this trial at any time.

Chapter 12
Health Care Teams:
The Importance of Experience and Volume

Many people have their routine health care needs met by going to their family doctor or to a medical clinic with which they are familiar. Your doctor or clinic may be accessible and convenient, and may be close to your home. These family doctors and the staff at clinics are frequently caring. They may know you well, have cared for your medical conditions over time, and thus can offer continuity for your ongoing health care. All are important factors in receiving good health care.

The way people initially choose their regular providers for their routine care differ widely. You may have chosen your doctor based on advice friends have given you. You may be continuing a pattern of many years of care in your family. The location may have been convenient, or making the first appointment was simple. Perhaps you were referred to this person by another health care provider. Sometimes it is just a coincidence which primary care provider you end up with, and sometimes your health insurance has a strong influence.

In this chapter, we'll consider times and situations that call for making a more considered or different choice of where to go and who you want to see for your care. This is of particular importance when you have complex medical conditions, have a rare (infrequently seen) medical condition, or are in need of highly technical medical services. There are several factors worth considering, in addition to convenience and familiarity and continuity of care, when making such a choice. They are:

- *Ongoing experience* leads to better outcomes. This refers to a person (or facility) that has extensive current experience in a particular technology, whether for diagnostic or therapeutic procedures. This is particularly important for complex procedures.
- As *volume* increases, the frequency of complications decreases. This refers to the number of particular diagnostic tests or surgical procedures or other interventions being performed in a medical center or by a particular team of providers each month or each year.
- Care by health care providers with more *current experience* in particularly complex conditions leads to longer survival and better quality of life.
- *Tertiary care centers,* where people are referred for complex or infrequent medical situations and conditions, have better results. The staff in these centers is well informed by new and evolving science.
- *Specialty institutions* merit consideration. These institutions focus on particular types of procedures, so their providers and teams of care givers have both volume and experience in their area of expertise.

Bob is 60 years old. Around dinner time one evening he developed severe squeezing chest pain and nausea. His wife, Helen, who is a nurse practitioner, recognized the symptoms as suspicious for a heart attack and called 911. The emergency medical system workers came promptly, took the appropriate initial measures, and immediately started to drive to the nearest community hospital. Helen strongly and clearly stated that they must take him to the main hospital center in their city, which would mean driving 20 extra minutes because she knew that this larger medical center had the facilities and experience to intervene urgently with patients having heart attacks. These interventions include cardiac (heart) catheterization and angioplasty. She was well informed as to the benefits of early intervention in people suffering from a heart attack and was also aware of where these services were available locally. These specialized services, if performed soon after the onset of the symptoms, can save lives and decrease the amount of heart damage for people having heart attacks.

This can result in an improved quality of life for the patients. These services can only be provided by experienced cardiologists, as part of a team that works in centers which have appropriate facilities.

Most people are not as well informed as Helen regarding the needs of patients having a heart attack, and the facilities that can provide the care. Bob had an angioplasty and stent placement promptly, which limited the damage to his heart, and has fully recovered. People who suffer acute vascular events, such as strokes and heart attacks, may benefit from urgent intervention by experienced staff at well-equipped hospitals. Most medical conditions do not require urgent intervention, so time is usually available to search for the best place to obtain the health care needed.

Surgery and Procedures

A variety of reviews of the outcome for patients who have undergone complex surgery have shown that were fewer complications, lower death rates, and more rapid recoveries when the surgeon and surgical team providing the services had greater experience in the procedures. (Examples of the complex surgeries in these reviews have included the repair of aortic aneurysms, hip replacements, cancer surgery, and transplantation procedures.) This experience was defined as *the number of surgeries per year* of the type being reviewed. In other words, recent experience and greater volumes of that experience improve the chances of success for that particular procedure. For example, one study compared total hip replacements and found that surgeons who performed more than 60 replacements per year had proportionally fewer complications than those who performed 30 or less. The definition of "experience" or "high volume" is different for different procedures. For example, there are many fewer heart transplants each year than hip replacements, so the opportunity to gain that experience is vastly different.

The effect of volume and experience is also seen in procedures such as heart surgeries and catheterizations, the placement of devices such as pacemakers or defibrillators, or the performance of angioplasty and the insertion of a stent. There is an understanding that volume and experience as factors include both the doctor leading the procedure and the team supporting this leader. This seems logical since teams tend to perform better when they have more practice in their particular "game" or activity. The centers that have greater experience in specialized procedures tend to report better outcomes than lower volume centers.

Emily is in her late 60's and has developed a condition called Dupuytren's contracture. In this condition, there is scarring of the tendons that move the last 3 fingers in her right (dominant) hand. It makes it difficult to grasp items tightly or to open her hand due to these scars. She consulted two hand surgeons, and each suggested a procedure to remove the scars, however, their suggestions were for significantly different surgeries. One involved three to four hours of invasive surgery and required months of recovery, the other was less complicated (one hour of invasive surgery) but still would require 8 or more weeks for her to recover and resume normal activities. She wondered why two similar specialists would recommend such different procedures for the same problem. Her research revealed that each of these procedures is considered reasonable by traditional hand-surgery groups in the U.S., with the more complex procedure having fewer recurrences of these contractures in the years after the surgery. But neither was risk-free. Both procedures involved opening the skin and operating directly on the tendon areas.

What was really interesting to Emily was the discovery of another much less invasive surgery where a fine or very thin needle is used to remove the scars without opening the skin. It was being offered in Europe and by several hand-surgery specialized centers in the U.S. The results being reported from this novel approach were encouraging. One U.S. clinic that she contacted told her they did more than 3,000 such procedures per year. The downside was that proportionally more people needed a second procedure in the future, due to a recurrence of the contractures. If there was a recurrence, this procedure could be repeated or the more traditional surgery performed. The cost was less than one-fifth of the more invasive approach, the recovery time was one-fifth as long, and there was less risk of complications from anesthesia and infections than the more complex procedures. It required travel to another state where the specialized center was located. Emily chose to have the fine needle procedure, and she recovered rapidly and resumed her tennis playing in a month. There has since been a gradual recurrence of the contracture, however, in the year after the procedure.

Results suggest that for many, but not all procedures, patients do better under the care of hospitals and physicians that perform that procedure frequently. This is a general statement, and there is some variation in the effect of experience in the outcomes. Physicians' and hospitals' skills may improve when they do procedures more often. Consider these factors when making a choice of where to have a procedure done. You should ask the following questions.

• How many of *these procedures* did you perform in the past year?
• How many were done in *this* medical center?
• What complications have occurred after the procedure?
• What is the *rate* of complications from this procedure?
• How many people have died last year (or in the last 2 years) as a result of undergoing this procedure?

A hospital information officer or a particular member of the team that does the procedure being considered should give you *specific* answers to these questions. Answers such as "many" or "frequent", or to the question on complications answers like "almost never" or "seldom", are not acceptable. Numerical answers to these questions can be compared from one center to another, and this information can be used as in making a choice.

Complex Medical Conditions

Similar considerations are relevant for patients with complex conditions. This has been seen clearly in the care of patients with HIV/AIDS. This is a relatively newly recognized complex medical condition, but with a rapidly evolving understanding of the basic science underlying the disease. There has been a rapid application of this new understanding in developing tests to check on the status of the patient, and treatments to control the condition. Knowledge of these developments has required active participation and collaboration among the physicians who are caring for patients with HIV/AIDS, in order to keep up with this rapid growth of information. New medications and monitoring approaches have clearly improved the quality of life and life expectancy of people with this disease. Integrating these scientific advances into the care of the patients was most effectively done by doctors who had larger numbers of patients they were working with. The *survival* and *well-being* of patients with AIDS is significantly associated with the *experience* in that disease of physicians who treat them. The greater the number of patients with AIDS that the physician had cared for, and that they were currently caring for, the longer their patients lived. Since AIDS is a relatively new disease and emerging research information is guiding its treatment, those centers with more patients (greater volume) have more ability to be informed of the new research and to fully utilize the results. The familiarity of the health care providers with the medications and the use of laboratory testing to guide treatment has made the care of their patients more efficient (used fewer tests, medicines, surgeries, less time in hospital), and more effective.

Connie has chronic lung disease as a result of many years of smoking. She now becomes breathless with very little activity. Her local doctor properly suggested she needed supplemental oxygen treatments, and obtained this for her. But she did not know when she should be using it, how to monitor how she was doing, and whether she might be able to improve her ability to be active by using other medications or by having training and exercise to be in better condition. She felt uncertain as to when she might be putting herself in danger and what was safe for her to do. Her doctor did not guide her in this, as he had limited experience with patients who were on supplemental oxygen.

Connie learned that the university medical center near her home had a specialized clinic for people with chronic lung disease, and had a rehabilitation program for such patients. She promptly enrolled in this program. She was prescribed new medications that make breathing easier, was introduced to an exercise program that carefully monitors her oxygen levels and heart responses to the exercise. She has learned how to continue this type of activity on her own. She has been taught how and when it is best to use the supplemental oxygen. She has been continuing the exercises on her own and has improved her physical condition and ability to remain active. She now feels much better and is more confident that she can manage her condition.

This effect of experience and volume has been noted among those who care for people with cancer, tuberculosis, and other severe medical conditions. Its effects have been seen in the care of patients in intensive care units who have heart failure, respiratory failure, and kidney diseases. Any time a person is hospitalized for a severe condition, clinicians experienced in *that condition* usually achieve better results. Since people are hospitalized less frequently than in the past, and now only for severe conditions, it can be valuable to consult experienced "hospitalists" (doctors who specialize in caring for patients in the hospital) who offer such services.

To be clear, this advice refers to *current and ongoing* experience and volume. This does not refer to *past* experience. Being older or having practiced medicine for a longer time can be valuable, but is not what is necessarily important. In fact, there are reviews that examined the relationship between the duration of clinical experience (number of years in practice) and performance. The results of these reviews suggest that older physicians who have been in practice for many years actually possess less factual knowledge, are less aware of the latest (cutting edge) science in medicine, are less likely to adhere to appropriate standards of care, and may also have poorer patient outcomes, than younger doctors in active practices. The health care providers with the best results were those associated with medical educational institutions. For these physicians, having been in practice for many years did not cause them to have poorer patient outcomes or less knowledge of recent advances in medical knowledge.

Tertiary or Referral Medical Centers

Consultations for complex or unusual medical conditions frequently take place in tertiary care centers. These are large medical centers which are often associated with educational institutions. They are called "tertiary" because patients may be referred to these after going to a primary care provider or to a local referral center (the secondary center). While going to such tertiary care institutions may be daunting, and may require travel away from home, they are worth considering for complex and unusual conditions and procedures. There is much new scientific knowledge published in a variety of medical journals and being discussed in various meetings of medical professional groups. Applying this new information to clinical care takes time and requires the team of providers to be absolutely up to date. For many busy practitioners, this is not possible. For those who teach medicine or who are involved in acquiring this information (being involved in research activities in their field), staying current is an essential part of their work. In particular situations such as the treatment of advanced cancers, AIDS, and newly identified conditions like tuberculosis that is resistant to antibiotics, choosing a doctor with cutting-edge knowledge in that field can lead to receiving cutting-edge care and better results.

Many people have stated that the convenience of a location near home, where family and friends can visit easily, and transportation is simple, is an important factor in their choice for obtaining medical care. Community health care providers and community hospitals offer valuable services, and for the great majority of our needs, the local health care facilities are more than adequate. It makes sense to be concerned about the disruption of familiar patterns and the comfort of being near home and near your community when deciding where to seek your health care. But there are times when other options give you the opportunity to improve the chances of meeting your health care needs, and having the best outcome possible.

Section 5

Personal Observations and Perspectives

This section differs from the previous four, in that the ideas presented are based on my own personal experiences and opinions, rather than on empirical evidence. Health care is partly based on science, partly on experience, partly on instincts, and partly on beliefs. Diagnoses and treatments are often imperfect. Decisions are made with some uncertainty.

Using high-quality evidence to make decisions improves the chances of good outcomes, but evidence that is directly applicable to a particular situation is not always available. When reliable evidence cannot be found to apply directly to a particular concern, it is reasonable to make deductions from the evidence available from similar situations, with the understanding that we cannot be certain that our conclusions are fully correct. When no clear scientific evidence can be found, "expert opinion" is another source of information that can help guide a decision. The opinions of such experts are based on their practice experience and their understanding of a body of knowledge. Experience and expert opinions are considered a form of evidence, though felt to be of a lesser quality as that based on studies utilizing scientific methodology.

In this section, I offer my perspective on situations you may find yourself in, which can affect the decisions you will make, the decisions the doctor makes, the relationships between doctors and patients as well as between patients, family, and friends. My hope is that giving you a broader view of these situations can help you recognize when you are in a similar one, and so be able to respond in a wiser and more satisfying fashion. Further, these chapters are my attempt to help you make choices in how you approach issues around health care, including the choice of a primary care doctor and the choice of how to be supported when you are involved in health care situations.

Personal Observation 1
The Forest and the Trees:
Treating the Numbers or Treating the Patient

When you have a periodic health review or appraisal, your doctor often looks at "markers" that are associated with risks to your health. For example, we may want to know what your cholesterol level is since high cholesterol raises the probability of a heart attack or stroke. High cholesterol is a "marker" for an increased chance of cardiovascular disease. You may have a bone density exam because low bone density increases the chance of having a fracture. A low bone density is a "marker" indicating increased chance for a future fracture. High blood pressure is a marker for increased likelihood of having kidney failure, having a stroke, and having heart failure. In people with HIV/AIDS, we follow the lymphocyte counts since a low CD4 lymphocyte count is a marker for a possible complication. We refer to these as **surrogate markers**. They provide information on the chances of a bad outcome we want to avoid. Since the outcome is an event which you will have or will not have, and cannot be measured otherwise (it is all or none), we substitute these measurements of the markers to give us more precise information on the probability of that bad outcome. But they are *not* the outcome.

These *surrogate markers* are usually easy to measure. Often we get very specific numerical results, such as for cholesterol level (in milligrams per 100 milliliters of blood) or blood pressure (for our systolic and diastolic pressures in millimeters of mercury). Patients frequently pay strict and close attention to these numbers. Doctors and patients set goals to improve the results of these markers, thus lowering the risk of a bad event. If you work hard to achieve these goals, you can be pleased if the results improve and may be upset if they do not.

It is worth remembering that each surrogate marker represents only one factor in the chance of having a bad outcome. There are other ways to lower the risk of a particular outcome that are not reflected in the measurements of individual markers. For example, smoking increases the probability of heart disease. Stopping smoking decreases this chance, but it does this without altering the cholesterol level or blood pressure measurements. There is no surrogate marker that informs how stopping smoking lowers the chances of a bad event. Observations over the last 50 years have clearly shown this to be the case, however.

Here is another example. A low bone density measurement, indicating osteoporosis, increases the chances of having a bone fracture. Yet an important risk for a fracture is falling. Preventing accidents in the home that may cause a fall (removing certain hazards around the house) has been shown to be a robust way of lowering the risks of a fracture, regardless of the bone density measurement.

Frank is infected with HIV. We measure his CD4 lymphocytes periodically, as a measure of the status of his immune system. This marker provides information on his risk of developing an infection. His mood is affected markedly by the results of his CD4 counts. When his value was 550, he was happy. The next measure was 510 and he was quite upset for a number of days. He felt very vulnerable. Yet, these numbers are quite similar and within the range of laboratory variations, as well as the measured variations that happen naturally in everyone with this condition from day to day. One day he told me that he started taking B vitamins because they might increase his lymphocyte counts. I reminded him that washing his hands and making sure his food was carefully prepared were important ways to lower the risks of infection, even though this cannot be measured like his lymphocytes can be. Getting the proper vaccines would probably also help. I wanted him to understand that his health behaviors, his habits, and overall approach to life were more important than a few laboratory tests. There are more trees than the surrogate marker which is his CD4 level, in his forest.

Joe is 52 years old. In a health appraisal, we measured his total cholesterol which was 242 and his HDL cholesterol which was 44. After his visit, he started a regular exercise program and changed his diet to reduce animal fats and trans fats, which he was quite disciplined in following. When he returned for a repeat exam after 3 months, he had lost 6 pounds, but his cholesterol was 231 and the HDL was 43 at that exam, hardly different. He was quite dispirited. I told him that populations that ate a healthy diet such as he now was eating (referred to as the Mediterranean diet), and were physically active, as he now was, had lower rates of heart problems than those that were sedentary and were not careful of what they ate, even when the cholesterol levels were the same! This meant that even with the minimal change in his surrogate marker (cholesterol) values, he had lowered his risks substantially by changing his lifestyle. The surrogate marker was an obvious tree, yet the forest was larger and more complex than the one tree he had been concentrating on.

It is easy to focus on an individual marker. They are *available,* appear to be very precise, and can be followed over time. It is important to remember, however, that *surrogate markers* are not the ultimate goal. Living better and longer is the ultimate goal. These markers may motivate people to change their habits and see whether the marker changes. However, the numerical values of these markers are only part of the story. There are many trees in your forest.

Personal Observations 2
Expectations

When I was in primary care practice, there were times when I thought that a patient I was seeing in my office wanted me to offer a treatment or a diagnostic test which I felt was not necessary or appropriate. Sometimes this pressure was articulated directly, such as the university executive mentioned in the *Prologue* who requested antibiotics for his sore throat. At other times it seemed more indirect, with perhaps body language or facial expressions that showed disappointment that I had no particular medications to recommend for their condition. There were times, however, when I thought the patient wanted me to recommend further diagnostic testing or to provide some treatment, and I was wrong.

One example was Sarah, a woman in her 20s. During the first visit, she described difficulties with having regular bowel movements, sometimes not defecating for several days, and then having 2 or 3 movements a day for several days. She also had cramping pains and loss of appetite. She had not lost weight, and these symptoms did not interfere with her sleep. I did a physical examination and ordered a blood test and a stool test looking for inflammation. When her exam and tests were normal, I explained that she probably had "irritable bowel syndrome", and it would be best to start a treatment program with a diet. We would observe her symptoms to see if they changed with the diet I proposed. I thought she would be unhappy that I was not offering her a medication to cure her condition. Instead, she said, "That is good news! I would rather avoid medicines if I can." Evidently, my initial expectations were based on some of my own internal reactions and feelings, not from communications from Sarah. I felt relieved by her response.

Doctors want patients to like them, and to be pleased with their approaches to their medical issues. We sometimes think that if a patient leaves our office "empty handed", with no plan to go to the laboratory for a diagnostic test or with no prescription, they will be disappointed. They took the time, effort, and expense to come for a medical visit, and did not leave with anything material. We may offer to run a test, just to make them feel that we are being thorough. We may offer a treatment to fulfill an expectation that we sense from them. Sometimes doctors will make suggestions to use medicines that are "over the counter", some of which are not known to be effective. There are cough syrups and expectorants for cold symptoms, and drugs to treat intestinal symptoms that do not have any proven benefit. This "generosity" from the medical provider does make some people feel they are being cared for, and that their concerns were taken seriously. There are times, however, when our expectations are wrong.

As I discussed in the "*More Care may not Necessarily be Better Care*" chapter in this book, these "gifts" from the doctor may not represent high-quality medical care. A gift from a person in authority is frequently accepted with gratitude. There is a feeling that they care about us. It is not easy to consider this objectively. These gifts are difficult to reject. However, advice, ideas, and information are also "something" to go home with. Written information about a condition or advice for lifestyle changes is also something tangible. When a doctor offers verbal explanations but no prescription, it can be considered a gift, and it is reasonable to be pleased at not being given unnecessary medicines or placebos. Observing a set of symptoms to see how they change during the day, or as we alter our activities, can be a useful diagnostic step. Keeping notes or a measure of these symptoms over time and with different activities is *doing something* that can provide useful information.

If a patient expresses appreciation to her doctor for the care she is receiving, including the times when no tests or prescriptions are recommended, this provides the doctor positive feedback. It allows the doctor to review his or her own expectations that patients want some sort of intervention each time they come to the office. It makes it more likely the doctor will offer an explanation or give the "good news" that no treatment is necessary. This can help free doctors to fulfill their desire to provide high-quality care.

Personal Observation 3
Support:
Often a Help, Sometimes a Hindrance

Having support when you have health care issues to deal with can facilitate the process of getting high-quality health care. Particularly when visiting health care providers, being accompanied by someone you trust can make the process easier and better. This includes ensuring that your agenda is fully expressed and heard when you go to see a health care provider. Having more than one person listening and asking questions increases the chances of understanding the information offered and the plans for the evaluation of your condition. It increases the chances that you will remember the goals of the treatments and the particular treatment instructions you must follow. It increases your confidence, ability to ask questions, and to express your preferences and opinions. The support you receive can provide time and space for you to think and respond to the situation, particularly if you are in discomfort or afraid. You can be supported and assisted by family members, close friends, or other advisors.

When you are facing a structured system that has a hierarchy where doctors have great authority, having support can provide you with the confidence and ability to maintain your autonomy. This allows you to participate in the decision making process. The traditional medical model is paternalistic and authoritarian. This is changing, as doctors cede authority and patients recognize their right to be active participants. Support augments this process.

Anna returned for a visit in my office nine months after she last came to see me. In the previous visit, she was accompanied by her mother. She is a 40-year-old woman whose initial complaints were muscle stiffness and muscular aches that had lasted over a period of about six months prior to the first visit. These pains were worse after she played tennis, which was an important part of her life, so she had stopped this activity. She had been sleeping poorly and feeling exhausted. Her exam on the initial visit revealed some tender spots on her back and chest. Her laboratory tests were normal.

She came for the return visit (the first visit after her initial evaluation) with her mother to discuss the diagnostic and treatment plans. I told her I thought she had a disorder (or syndrome) called "fibromyalgia", and offered several options for treatment. These included medications which help restore normal sleep and modulate pain, and a moderate exercise program when she started feeling better. Alternatively, I offered to refer her to a clinic which specialized in fibromyalgia in a nearby academic medical center. During this return visit, Anna's mother had asked if I felt nutritional therapy and acupuncture would be a better approach for this problem. I told them I had not seen any evidence that this approach was effective. Her mother assured me that a friend of hers with a similar problem had seen a "nutriologist" who had given her friend a therapeutic diet. This friend also had a series of acupuncture sessions and felt improved. She thought her daughter should try this approach first since it seemed more "natural" to her. I informed Anna that the insurance was unlikely to pay for these alternative treatments. I suggested that we should review her progress in a few months, and she could report which treatment she had tried and their effectiveness. I reinforced the idea that observation and charting her response to treatments and lifestyle changes would be a useful diagnostic step as well as potentially therapeutic for her condition.

In this return visit nine months later, Anna came alone. She told me she had received 10 acupuncture treatments in the time since the last visit with her mother. She had also been seeing her nutriologist regularly and following the therapeutic diet prescribed, and had taken nutritional supplements that her nutrition specialist had prescribed for her. She felt no better. She had spent $2,500 on these treatments and now wanted to try my treatment recommendations. Over the next six months, Anna took a medication I prescribed and gradually started an exercise program. Her symptoms lessened over time. She is now back playing doubles tennis. The initial, strong advice from Anna's mother was given with good intentions. Yet it was based on "available" information that confirmed beliefs around health care for both of them and created several shortcuts to critical decision making.

Support often comes from family members. Parents frequently take the responsibility for making decisions for their children, and even as the children become adults, they continue to be involved in this manner. As children grow older, they gradually become independent of the parents and more autonomous. Often, however, some remnants of this paternalistic relationship remain. Parents want the best for their children, want to fix whatever problems they may have, and may have strong opinions on what is best for them. Voicing these strong opinions or beliefs can interfere with critical decision making as I described in Section 1. If we have a paternalistic supporter in dealing with the health care structure, we may be caught in the middle of the doctor's authority and our supporter's views, between the two authorities. This makes it more difficult for us to feel autonomous and to feel confident in critically considering the choices we are facing, and to fully participate in making informed choices.

Constructive and helpful support gives the patient comfort and confidence. It helps the patient fully express her agenda to the doctor. Patients and companions can ask questions if they attend medical visits together. This support promotes the ability of the patient and supporter to pay full attention to the discussion with the doctor. It promotes careful consideration of all information and options. Consideration of the options can be done with the doctor or after the visit with the doctor, or both.

If the support is authoritarian and based on beliefs, it can create an antagonistic situation with the doctor, who may also tend toward paternalism, particularly if the support person and the doctor disagree.

Alternatively, strong support, when it is in agreement with the doctor's views, puts more pressure on a patient to follow this advice and makes it difficult for her to carefully consider other options.

Support may come from family members, including parents, adult children, and siblings. It may come from friends. Support may come from professional sources, such as advocates, social workers, and religious community members. It can include accompanying the patient to visits with the health care provider. Helping with preparing for visits or consideration of the results of the visit can also be further supportive activities. At different points in this book, I have suggested that having support is an important strategy for participating fully in making "informed choices". This strategy supports careful decision making to help you avoid pitfalls and shortcuts in making a choice. Choosing the best source of support is a consequential decision we must make.

Personal Observation 4
Caregivers Need Support Too

Providing support for people we care about can be a gratifying experience. Being generous with your time and energy is a virtue, and can provide a sense of well-being and satisfaction. Participating in care giving and support can also provide you with the comfort of knowing that you can also receive support in a situation where you may need it. However, being a care giver may also cause difficulties.

Pat came to see me on a routine visit to follow-up on his high blood pressure treatment. As soon as he entered my office, I could see he was distressed, and I asked him what was concerning him. He told me his wife, Joan, had been diagnosed with a type of leukemia, and he was frightened. She was facing treatments with powerful medications lasting several months. While the chances to control her disease were good, she faced a prolonged period of feeling weak and quite sick, and of being vulnerable to infections and other complications as a result of her treatment. He was planning to reduce his work to part-time in order to be able to give her the appropriate care and support, and to make sure she had the food and comforts she might need. She was being very brave, he told me, and he was afraid that his fears would be apparent and upset her.

I discussed with him the importance of maintaining his health and energy during this time. For him to be able to provide the support Joan would need, he needed to take care of his own needs as well. I discussed with him my observations of how difficult it is for us when people we care about are sick. We may not want to reveal our anxieties and fears since that may make the sick person feel worse. We may feel tired or bored, even irritated at times, from the stress and duties of care-taking. It may interfere with our sleep and rest. We can feel burdened by the work and responsibility of being a care giver. This makes us feel worse and even guilty since we are not the ones who are sick and suffering. When the illness is prolonged, and when the chances of improvement are not good, these uncomfortable feelings are exacerbated. The physical strain can accumulate and exhaust us.

Many studies have documented stress, depression, and a sense of burden among care givers. This has been noted particularly among persons caring for patients with dementia and after a person suffers a stroke. It has also been seen in people caring for older patients who are frail and bedridden or terminally ill. The well-being of care givers suffers as the length of the disability of the person being cared for increases, and when the disability is more severe. Depression in care givers gradually declines in intensity after the person they were caring for has died, though it can still be a problem a year later.

I scheduled Pat for a return visit in a month's time, to make certain that his blood pressure control did not suffer during the stress of Joan's treatments. I also wanted to be able to assess the burden and distress he was feeling as Joan's treatments progressed. When he returned, he readily described his difficulties in sleeping. He had also been irritable with some of the people who visited Joan. They always seemed to have suggestions about how her care might be improved, which he saw as a criticism of his care. He had not had much time to relax, nor to concentrate on his own work. He felt guilty in wanting to get away from the house and play golf. Joan continued to be courageous and unafraid.

I asked Pat what other resources he had available to help him with Joan's care. She did have good friends who were willing to spend time with her. There were community members who offered to provide meals at times, yet, he had felt unwilling to "impose" on them. After a discussion, he accepted that he would be more patient and less burdened if he had some time off. He would appreciate the opportunity to go to work, at times. I also pointed out that there were people who cared about both Joan and him, who would feel good at having the opportunity to help. I also suggested that Joan might appreciate a variety of companionship, and might just be glad to be free of his company from time to time!

The next month, when he returned, he was feeling much better. Joan was still frail and vulnerable from her treatments, yet, she remained hopeful and courageous. Pat had established a schedule of helpers to give him time off from those responsibilities. There had also been some meals provided. Some of the care was being provided by professional home helpers from a local agency. He had, in turn, become less irritable, more energetic, and more patient.

The burden and stress on care givers and supporters can be considerable. Care giver depression can be severe and may require clinical treatment. Support for the supporters can provide them the respite needed to be able to continue to be effective and competent in the care they are providing. To receive support requires the supporter to acknowledge his or her own needs and to accept well-intentioned offers of assistance.

Personal Observation 5

Choosing a Primary Care Physician

In television advertisements in 1993, Harry and Louise sat at their kitchen table talking, claiming that the health care reforms proposed by the Clinton Administration were going to take away the freedom of Americans to choose their personal physicians. These advertisements, which were funded by health insurance companies, are believed to have been influential in defeating those proposals in 1994. The Affordable Care Act of 2010 did not change the ability of Americans to choose their doctors. The concept of freedom to choose your personal doctor is important to Americans. In fact, how free are you in your choice of primary care physician?

In many cases, the choice of who you can see as a primary care provider is quite limited. Your health insurance plan may limit your choices to doctors who participate in your plan. You may be assigned to a particular primary care provider by your health insurance plan. If you get your health care through the Veterans Administration Medical System, then you can see only doctors who work for them. The millions of Americans without health insurance go mainly to clinics that serve medically indigent people or go to emergency-care clinics, hence often have little choice in selecting their primary care provider.

If you do have some freedom to choose your doctors, how carefully and how often do you exercise that freedom? Even when choices are possible, people frequently don't select carefully among the available possibilities. Often, people continue to see one physician for a long time, even if they are not fully satisfied with the care they are receiving. The *preference for the status quo* (Chapter 3) is one factor that inhibits switching to a different doctor. When people do need to make a choice, they are often influenced by *heuristics* or shortcuts in making decisions (Section 1), such as basing the choice on the experience of a relative or friend, or perhaps on an article providing popular ratings among local physicians (which are usually influenced by public relations agencies), rather than basing the choice on a set of logical criteria.

When I left my primary care practice, many of my patients asked me for advice about which doctor might serve them best in my place. I have also been asked for the same advice in my work as a patient advocate, and by friends and family. I have also had to make similar choices for myself. I looked for evidence that would help guide my recommendations but was unable to find any scientific articles that provided particular characteristics of primary care doctors which led to improved health care quality or outcomes among their patients. As far as I can determine, such studies have not been done.

Since I wanted to be able to give advice based on objective criteria, I thought about what characteristics would seem logical to evaluate in choosing a doctor, even if there is no empirical evidence supporting these. Based on my experience and observations over the years of medical practice and patient advocacy work, I have prepared a list of criteria that I feel are important to consider when choosing a personal doctor who will be more likely to provide high-quality medical care. You may not be able to consider all of these characteristics, but I think this list can provide an objective approach to help you make a sound choice of a primary care doctor. I have also developed "red flags", or characteristics that I think are reasons for rejection of a particular choice. The list may even help you decide that it is time to change your doctor.

Medical Ethics: A doctor must be impeccable in following the principles of medical ethics. The patient's well-being and best interests must be in the forefront of the doctor's considerations. Any conflict of interest which can interfere with this is a red flag. Promoting products, particularly if they are available through the doctor's office, is an example of a red flag. There are doctors who have investments in laboratories where they send patients to have tests done or have pharmacies in their offices where they sell medications and supplies to their patients. This creates financial incentives to do more tests or to provide more medications, which are questionable practices. Equipment for performing specialized tests in the office (and owned by the practice) can be a convenience to both the doctors and their patients, but their use must be considered scrupulously. It is reasonable for you to receive a clear and logical answer to the question: How can this test help guide my treatment? Honesty is an essential characteristic of an ethical medical practitioner.

Your doctor must respect your autonomy, one of the principles of medical ethics. You have a right to participate in making medical decisions, and in this book I have described how making informed choices improves the quality of your health care. If a doctor diminishes your ability to make choices or does not give you the time and space, doesn't listen or provide the information you need to participate in making decisions in your health care, those failures are a red flag.

Reputation: How the doctor is regarded by his peers in the medical community provides helpful information. Doctors work in collaboration with other physicians, sometimes consulting with them, at other times sharing ideas at meetings and educational events. Their peers will have opinions on the attitudes, knowledge, and clinical judgment that the doctor exhibits. They may also express opinions on their colleague's personality or style that is worth listening to. Doctors may not be willing to give critical information about a peer, so you will need to listen carefully to evaluate how enthusiastic their positive statements are and to detect any nuances in the information provided.

Friends or family members who have some experience with the doctor can also provide useful information. How likable they are is not the important concern. But if some of the comments suggest a lack of respect for their patients, failure to listen to their patients, lack of follow-through with plans, or being inconsiderate, these are red flags of caution. Information from people who you know and who have experience with a doctor on key characteristics such as accessibility, reliability, and personality can be useful.

I have seen articles in magazines in listing the ten best doctors in each particular specialty in the local area. I consider this to be a publicity stunt both for the magazine and some doctors. The criteria needed to make it into one of these lists amount to nothing more than a popularity contest, and I don't think this the proper measure of the quality of the health care they provide.

Relationship to you: You want your doctor to be fully objective in his or her evaluation and recommendations for you. *This is not possible if he or she is a family member or a close friend.* When personal boundaries are blurred and the role as a personal physician is combined with another relationship, then the doctor's personal anxieties and fears can interfere with his or her judgment. The doctor may fear giving bad news and hence deny in his or her own mind any possible serious problems. Alternatively, anxiety and the desire to be a good friend may make the doctor unable to realistically consider a serious diagnosis to be very improbable, and, therefore, order extensive and possibly unnecessary testing to see if it is the correct diagnosis. There is a saying in medicine, "If you hear hoofbeats, don't look for zebras." This refers to overzealous searches for improbable diagnoses. The more common possibilities should be eliminated first. When doctors prescribe diagnostic tests in trying to confirm the presence or absence of an improbable disease, it incurs a cost, takes time and effort, may pose risks, and causes anxiety. Fears and anxieties that doctors have about a patient are also contagious. The patient becomes more afraid and anxious, too.

If you feel that the doctor does not like you, that is a red flag. Negative feelings for a patient can influence a doctor's ability to carefully listen, to be patient, and to be thorough in the care of a patient. It is difficult to act beneficently to a person you dislike. Similarly, if a doctor expresses fondness in any manner that seems inappropriate, that crosses a relationship boundary and is a red flag.

Cultural Competence: We are characterized by diverse values, beliefs, behaviors, and experiences. Language differences exist. Our race, ethnic background, religion, gender identity, sexual preference, and age can cause difficulties in communicating with health care providers. Sensitivity to our particular cultural needs is important in being able to share intimate information in an understandable manner. The social, cultural, and linguistic needs individuals have for effective cross-cultural communication with their health care providers is another factor to consider in choosing a primary care provider. Barriers based on cultural differences can reduce the quality of health care provided.

Reputation among our communities for sensitivity to our special cultural need or identity as well as about language skills is one way of exploring this. Organizations that advocate for particular populations may have information on these skills and sensitivities. Some organizations provide cultural competency training and can provide information on professionals they have trained. An example of this for the LGBT community is SAGE (Services and Advocacy for Gay, Lesbian, Bisexual and Transgender Elders; http://sageusa.care/). The physician's office should answer direct questions as to the level of comfort and training in diverse populations. Can they communicate in the language that you speak? This does not mean the physician *must* be of the same ethnic background, gender, race, or ethnicity as you. But they must be accepting and welcoming and not judgemental towards your values, beliefs, identity, and needs.

Thoroughness: High-quality medical practice requires doctors to be complete in their examination and evaluation of patients. Not asking if you have an allergy to medications when giving a prescription is an example of not being thorough. I have seen doctors listen to lungs or hearts through clothing which impedes hearing abnormal lung or heart sounds. Other doctors do not take a temperature when a patient has other symptoms of an infection. Those are shortcuts or omissions that are red flags. The doctor must pay careful attention to your history and your physical exam.

Medical records must also be complete and up to date. Past visits, illnesses, hospitalizations, medications, and previous laboratory test results, must be recorded and easily accessed. *If a doctor does not keep records, it is not possible to have adequate continuity in your care, and it is a red flag.* You can see whether the doctor has your record available on each visit. Nowadays the record is often on a computer, but it should be available, and the doctor can refer to it during the visit. If your doctor has referred you to another physician, he should have shared appropriate information with the doctor he referred you to so he can have this available when you see him. You can also request a copy of your record for your own files at home, and have an opportunity to be sure the record is complete and up to date. The physician's office should not pose barriers for you in obtaining these records.

Reliability: Doctors must follow through with their plans for your care, and their staff must be trained to do likewise. If a doctor says he will send a prescription, request a laboratory test for you, or send you results of an evaluation, you expect him to do this.

Joe went to an orthopedist after he had suffered an ankle fracture. The day of his return visit he was to go first to the radiology office to have the ankle x-rayed. The orthopedist's staff had said that the request for this test would be at the radiology office when he arrived, yet it was not. He had to drive to the doctor's office, pick up the radiologist request, and go back to the radiology office to have the x-ray taken. He thought this inconvenience to him was due to a simple mistake. Yet when he had a return visit to get his walking boot, it had not been ordered, though he had been assured it would be. On a third occasion, the promised test request had not been completed and sent to the laboratory as he had been assured it would be, resulting in another inconvenience to him. This was not just one mistake. This was a pattern of not following through with small but important steps in a patient's care. This is an example of a red flag on reliability.

Personality: While being warm and likable are not characteristics I feel are imperative if a doctor is to provide high-quality health care, there are some personality traits that are important to consider in your choice of a doctor. She must be respectful and courteous. The doctor must be able to listen to your concerns and preferences with some patience. And she should be able to express her reasoning clearly about her concerns and plans she is considering for you.

If a doctor seems too self-important, too interested in how impressive he is, in your opinion of him, these are red flags. People overly invested and involved in their own ego can have a difficult time hearing other's opinions and concerns, since these can be interpreted as threats. You will have a difficult time being a participant in "informed choice" in your health care under those circumstances.

If a doctor is dismissive of your request for a second opinion, that is a red flag. Doctors should welcome the opportunity to have confirmation of their opinions or to learn from new perspectives that colleagues may offer. Lewis was being seen by a urologist for a bladder cancer. When he requested another opinion regarding the recommended treatment, the doctor dismissed the request as expressing disrespect and doubts about his care. This was a red flag for Lewis.

Accessibility: I value being able to reach my doctor to state my concerns or my questions. If the doctor does not respond promptly, this is a red flag. The doctor can inform you of the best way to reach her, perhaps email or telephone messages are the preferred methods. Today questions can be placed through telephone calls, emails, and increasingly through secure web access portals. But a response to your non-urgent questions should be provided within a few days, even if the response is that they cannot answer you fully at this time because they are busy or on vacation (an automated response or a response from a staff member informing you of this suffices).

There may be other factors that are important to you, personally. These can include a gender preference, the age of the physician, ethnic background, sensitivity to your cultural experiences, a pleasant and uncluttered waiting area, or a convenient office location. While these are characteristics that you should consider, they should not cause you to overlook the previously listed ones.

Marvin and I know each other from playing squash regularly. He had been assigned a primary care physician seven years before when he joined the local HMO as an employee of the university. Knowing that I am a doctor, he had complained to me about his doctor a number of times, over the years. The nature of his complaints seemed significant to me. We had talked about his changing to another primary care provider, but he had never made the change because it seemed too complicated to make a choice, to get to know the new doctor, and to have his records transferred.

Marvin had been driving a six-year-old car when he told me he had decided to buy a new one to replace it. He had thought about the type of vehicle that would best suit his needs and the features he would want it to have. He researched the prices of vehicles in that class and reviewed consumer buying guides. He looked at the frequency of repair records since he wanted a reliable car, and he also checked the safety test results and fuel efficiency of these vehicles. Finally, he went to the different dealers to test drive the three vehicles he had decided he would choose from.

I told him that it seemed paradoxical how much time and effort he put into choosing his new car. I compared it with his lack of effort in finding a more compatible physician and so improving the quality of the relationship he had with his doctor, and improve the quality of the health care he was receiving. He had been seeing his current doctor for longer than he had been driving the car he was replacing! Marvin is not unusual. Many people choose items to purchase with more care than they choose their doctors, even though the doctor who provides your primary care can have a profound impact on your life.

Choosing a primary care doctor is one of the health care decisions you may have to make. Making any such decisions wisely is not simple or easy. It requires time and careful considerations of your options. You will need to obtain reliable information, be willing to ask questions of people in positions of authority, and consult with trusted supporters and professionals. You must be able to listen openly and critically to the information and advice you are given. Making good decisions can improve your health care, the quality of your life, and even how long you will live

Epilogue

Collaboration*: working together toward common goals*

Craig called to tell me that when he first urinated that morning, the urine in the toilet bowl appeared cloudy. He knew that was not normal. I told him that cloudy urine sometimes is due to blood and protein being present, which would be considered abnormal, so we should examine his urine to see if this was the case. When his sample was analyzed later that day, there were red blood cells in his urine. This meant that we needed to search for the source of the blood by running some diagnostic tests. The next day he had a kidney x-ray exam, and this showed a tumor in his right kidney, which was the probable source of the bleeding into the urine.

Craig was a retired medical scientist from the university. His current activities included family events, playing tennis and golf, and an active involvement in community activities. I had always been impressed with his sharp wit, his logical approach to issues, and his clear and direct style of communicating. We had a working relationship that had started more than 20 years before.

He understood that this tumor could be a serious medical problem. He had a scan of his chest and abdomen as well as other routine tests which were normal. Surgery was scheduled for ten days after these tests. His right kidney was removed, and a cancer of the collecting system of that kidney was found. This cancer had begun to invade the normal tissue in that area of the kidney.

The oncologists (cancer specialists) told him that the best treatment for this type of cancer was surgical removal, which had just been performed. This did not guarantee, however, that the cancer had not already spread into other areas, even if there was no visible evidence. He faced about a 40% chance that there was microscopic spread that

194

would show up within the next two to three years. His type of cancer was resistant to radiation, and not very sensitive to chemotherapy. However, in view of the substantial chance of early spread, he was offered adjuvant chemotherapy, which entails using anti-cancer drugs to treat presumptive cancer cells prior to their becoming a visible tumor. He was told that there were no studies that evaluated adjuvant chemotherapy treatment for his particular tumor, but it had been shown to decrease the spread and growth of other types of tumors, such as breast and lung cancer. Since his type of cancer was fairly resistant to medications, however, the theoretical chance of being helpful was low.

Craig chose not to be treated presumptively. He said that for a small chance of benefit, he would certainly face serious adverse effects of the medications. He reminded me that Hippocrates had taught that we should not unduly burden the patient with our treatments. He said that if there was clear evidence of improved outcomes, he might consider it, but not simply based on the theory of possible benefit.

After two years of surveillance, no new tumors were seen. At the end of the third year, however, a scan revealed a tumor near his spine, an area that had been painful in the recent period. The biopsy of this tumor showed it to be a metastasis of his original cancer. The oncologist offered a course of chemotherapy. This would be given once every four weeks for six cycles. He informed Craig that the published observations on the effect of chemotherapy on his type of cancer showed some benefit. In comparing treatment to no treatment, patients lived an average of 3 months longer if treated. Those not treated survived an average of 6-8 months, with very rare patients living more than 12 months. Of those that were treated, about 5% lived more than two years.

Craig discussed this option with me extensively. He knew that the treatment would make him feel terrible. He would loose his hair. He would have aches and pains and nausea for 10 to 14 days following each treatment. He would gradually feel better over the next 10 to 14 days only to start again with the next cycle. He felt that spending six months of such poor quality of life only to gain three months was, in reality, losing three months of good quality of life. When I reframed the outcome to a five in 100 (or 1 in 20) chance of surviving more than two years, he responded that the odds were too low for him to take the gamble. I then showed him a graphic representation (figure below) of the chance of surviving more than two years. He responded that it seemed to him that the chance of survival looked very low and reminded me that every one of the 100 in the graphic that was treated with chemotherapy would suffer from the severe side effects of the treatment, and it would even possibly lead to the death of some. The choice he was making reflected his feelings of satisfaction that he had fulfilled all his responsibilities to his family, and that he had lived a full life. Now that he was retired, he felt free to let his life unfold without any heroic efforts to prolong it.

Figure

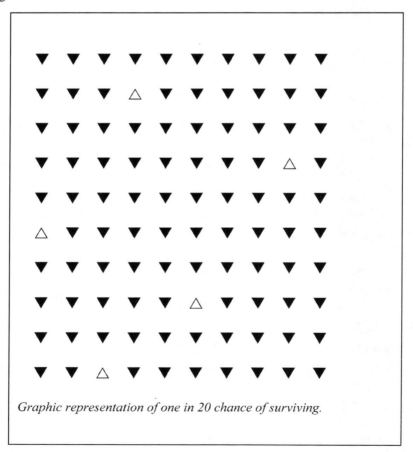

Graphic representation of one in 20 chance of surviving.

After it was clear that he understood the consequences of his choice, I suggested he speak with his family about this. His wife and daughter were very sad but were supportive of his decision. They knew he had thought about this and had come to a logical decision with which he was comfortable. His son, however, was very upset. He told Craig he felt it was a selfish decision, that he was not considering the effect on his family and his relationships. His son was planning to have a child, and he told Craig he had always yearned for his child to have a relationship with his grandfather.

This strong and intense reaction surprised Craig. His son had never been open with his feelings. Craig feared his son would feel resentful of his decision long after his death. Yet, he really did not want to have chemotherapy. It did not fit with the way he wanted to spend six months of the last period of his life. I wondered if there was another option to consider. Maybe there was a way of assessing the effect of the chemotherapy after one or two cycles so that he could stop the treatment if it appeared ineffective, or continue it if it appeared to be having the desired effect. This would show his son that he was making an effort to treat the cancer, and he could limit the undesired treatment if it did not have much chance of success.

Craig thought this might be a reasonable compromise. It fit with the Hippocratic mandate of considering the burden of treatments. He asked me to accompany him when he visited his oncologist with this question. The specialist felt it to be a reasonable strategy. If the cancer had shrunk by 50% or more after two cycles of chemotherapy, there was a chance that it would help control it. If the cancer did not shrink by at least that amount, then the treatment could be stopped, because there was no chance of it being helpful.

Craig went ahead with this plan. He had the expected severe adverse effects of the treatments, being virtually bedridden for the two weeks following each course of treatment, and felt quite weak the rest of the time. Prior to the third treatment, he had a scan that showed the tumor to be unchanged in size. He stopped the treatments. His family rallied around him, including his son. Six months later, the cancer had spread to his lungs, and he died at home after a month of hospice care. He had the satisfaction of having the understanding, love, and support of his family and friends. An unanticipated satisfaction was that the oncologist told him they would offer this option of assessing the early response of these tumors early in chemotherapy treatments to future patients, in order for them to make an informed choice to continue treatments or cease the therapy.

The collaboration between Craig, the oncologist, and I was satisfying for all. It led to carefully considered choices. It led to creating new options by our discussing the possibilities. I was not ill at ease as I had been with Professor Nwango (the case discussed in the Prologue), about the choices in management and treatment that Craig made in concert with the rest of his health care team. Craig felt satisfied that his preferences were carried out. While he altered his initial plans, this was due to family considerations. His family was satisfied with his choices and with the process. He and his son had no unresolved issues at the end of Craig's life. It was an example of an informed choice that considered personal values, life situation, and scientific evidence in reaching a decision.

This narrative of Craig's experiences illustrates how informed choice can lead to good health care decisions for an individual situation. Craig was an effective and active participant. He had the courage and ability to be clear about his preferences and values. He was able to obtain the information he required to carefully weigh his options. He participated with his health care providers in making decisions. The fundamental principles of medical ethics were respected. His autonomy was maintained and valued. Beneficence and non-maleficence were weighed in the decision making process. The principle of justice was also maintained by carefully choosing resources and treatments and by avoiding their misuse. It is my goal that the material presented in this book will make it more likely for readers like you to have satisfying experiences in obtaining the best health care available.

Supplementary Material

1. Medical Terminology

2. Risk Calculators

3. Going to the Doctor—How to be Prepared

4. Questions to Ask Regarding the Appropriateness of Care

5. Website Table

6. Advance Directives Tables

7. Living Will

8. Durable Power of Attorney

9. Do Not Resuscitate Order

1) Medical Terminology

The language used by your doctor to talk about your state of health and needs can be difficult to understand. This "medicalese" is gradually learned as doctors go through their training. It becomes the natural language that they use in describing medical conditions and symptoms, parts of the body, medication use, medical diagnostic tests, physical appearances, medical procedures and treatments, and any other scientific aspects of the care he or she may want to describe. It is really like a foreign language to most individuals. This language is frequently used in medical journals and medical textbooks as well. When the manuscript of this book was being reviewed, I was shown many examples of my use of medical terminology which would be difficult for the average reader to understand unless I translated it into common English. I needed non-medical reviewers to notice this.

In order to take a more active role in your health care, you will need to understand this medical terminology better. There are tools that help non-medical people translate this medical language into plain English. One useful tool is a website from *MedicineNet* that gives you these definitions on-line at http://www.medicinenet.com/medterms-medical-dictionary/article.htm.

There are also dictionaries that define medical terminology in common English. One is called **Webster's New World Medical Dictionary** (the third edition was released in 2008). Another more concise dictionary is the **Merriam-Webster's Medical Dictionary, New Edition** published in 2016.

2) Risk Calculators

There are formulae or "instruments" that you can use to calculate the probability of having a particular health event such as a heart attack or developing breast cancer in the future. These tools are based on studies in which large numbers of individuals were observed over many years. Based on the events or diseases from which these individuals suffered, factors associated with a probability of having the event were assessed and formulae developed for general use. These are available through internet sites where you enter your information on the web page, and the calculator computes the probability for your having a specific disease or event over the next several years.

Cardiovascular Disease Calculator

There is a calculator for the *probability of having a heart attack including dying from it in the next ten years*. This is based on the Framingham Study which followed the population of Framingham, Massachusetts over more than four decades. The *risk calculator* developed from this study has proven to be very robust in giving good estimates of risk and was validated through other similar studies. It is available through the internet at
http://cvdrisk.nhlbi.nih.gov/calculator.asp

To use this tool to calculate your probability of having a heart attack or death from a heart attack in the next ten years, you enter the following information:
- Your age in years
- Male or female sex
- Total Cholesterol level (an average of at least two measurements)
- HDL Cholesterol level (an average of at least two measurements)

- Smoker (any cigarette smoking in the last month, or non-smoker—yes or no)
- Latest Systolic Blood Pressure (the higher of the two numbers in a blood pressure reading)
- Are you currently on any medication to treat high blood pressure (yes or no)

The tool will calculate the percentage of people with your characteristics who will have a heart attack or die from coronary artery disease in the next ten years. For example, a 60-year old man who does not smoke, has a total cholesterol of 280, HDL-cholesterol of 48 and systolic blood pressure of 135, is not on medicines, and a is non-smoker has a ten-year risk of a heart attack or death from coronary disease of 14%. This means that on average, of 100 such men, 14 will have one of those events. If this man takes medications (such as a statin) to lower the cholesterol to 180 without any other changes in his values, his risk is lowered to 9% or 9 in 100 such men. This means that if 100 men take the medication over ten years, 5 heart attacks or deaths from coronary disease will have been prevented. Another way of framing the benefit of this intervention is that 20 men need to take the medication for ten years to prevent one event. (This is one way this risk calculator can be used.)

Breast Cancer

A *risk calculator* for breast cancer has been developed by scientists from the National Cancer Institute. This calculator is available through the internet at
http://www.cancer.gov/bcrisktool/Default.aspx.

This tool was designed to be used by health professionals so they would to be able to evaluate your personal risk of breast cancer and discuss this with you. It is, therefore, best to use this calculator in a conversation with your doctor. It is not applicable to any woman who already has had breast cancer.

The information needed to obtain a result includes:

- Do you have a history of any breast cancer or of ductal carcinoma *in situ* (DCIS) or lobular carcinoma *in situ* (LCIS)? If the answer is yes, then the tool will *not* provide a risk calculation.
- What is your age? (The tool is only for women 35 years of age or older)
- How old were you at the time of your first menstrual period?
- How old were you at the time of your first live birth of a child? (the answer is either no child or your age when your first child was born)
- How many first-degree relatives (mother, sisters, and daughters) have had breast cancer?
- Have you ever had a breast biopsy?
- If you have had a breast biopsy, how many total biopsies (positive or negative) have you had?
- If you had a biopsy, did you have a result that showed "atypical hyperplasia"? (This is a benign condition where cells look abnormal under the microscope but are not cancerous.)
- What is your race or ethnicity? (White, African-American, Hispanic, Asian or Pacific Islander, American-Indian or Alaskan-Native, other)

This calculator gives the risk of having or developing an invasive breast cancer over the next five years, and also provides the risk for a woman of the same age and ethnicity from the general U.S. population for comparison (a woman who would have answers to the above questions regarding age at first menstrual period, age at the first childbirth, etc. that is "average" for US women). For example, an average-risk white 63-year old woman has a risk of developing breast cancer in the next 5 years calculated at 1.9%. This means that 98.1% will *not* develop an invasive breast cancer in the next five years. Another way of stating this is that of 1,000 average white 63-year old women in the United States, 19 will develop an invasive breast cancer in the next five years and 981 will not.

Stroke Risk Calculator

A **stroke risk calculator** estimates your probability of having a stroke in the next 10 years. This information is also based on the Framingham Study and uses the following information:
- Sex
- Age
- Systolic Blood Pressure if you are not on medication for high blood pressure, or
- Systolic Blood Pressure if you are on a medication to treat high blood pressure
- Do you have diabetes?
- Are you a cigarette smoker?
- History of heart attack (myocardial infarction), coronary heart disease, angina pectoris or congestive heart failure (yes or no)
- History of atrial fibrillation (a type of heart rhythm irregularity)
- Do you have left ventricular hypertrophy (thickening of the heart muscle)?

The result from this tool will be the percentage of individuals with the same information that you provide that will have a stroke in the next ten years, or how many of 100 similar people will have a stroke after ten years. This is available at
http://www.stroke-education.com/calc/risk_calc.do

Other Risk Calculators

There are other tools. It is recommended they be used by heath care providers since the information that is used in these calculators requires some test results and answers to other medical questions which may require translation and extensive information on your past medical history.

A calculator for a **hip or other fracture** using bone mineral density as well as individual factors including gender, age, race/ethnicity, past medications and diagnoses, height and weight, family history, alcohol

consumption, and smoking is available at
http://www.shef.ac.uk/FRAX/

A calculator for the risk of **death from heart failure** has been developed. It is recommended that this tool be used with your healthcare provider since it requires information on types of medications being used to treat heart failure, laboratory data, and other sophisticated personal data that your doctor can provide clear answers for. The result it offers is the chance of surviving over the next one year, two years, and five years, as well as the average survival time for a person with your identical conditions.
This is available at *http://depts.washington.edu/shfm/index.php*

3) Going to the Doctor-How to be Prepared

Going to the Doctor-How to be Prepared

Plan:
1-**Goals**: list them in writing to take with you to the visit. Think about these for a few days prior to the visit and gather this list. Talk about this with family members and friends.

2-**Ideas and information**: bring information and sources to share and discuss.

3-**Support**: find a companion to come with you. This can be a family member (parent, child, sibling), trusted friend, professional advocate. This person should be aware of all your goals. The companion should understand their role such as taking notes, assuring that all your questions are all asked, that the instructions and plans from the doctor are clear and understood.

Prepare the doctor:
If possible, inform the doctor in advance of the questions and concerns that led to your wanting the visit are, if possible. This can be via regular mail, email, or telephone message.

During the visit:
Take notes or ask if taping the discussion of the visit is appropriate. Decide who will be the note taker or handle the taping.

Ask how to find out results of diagnostic tests like blood tests, x-ray exams, etc. Ask how you can inform the doctor if unanticipated reactions or symptoms develop from medications or from the condition(s) you are having evaluated and treated. What are the follow-up plans? Is there to be a return visit, if so when?

4) Questions to Ask Regarding the Appropriateness of Care

Questions Regarding the Appropriateness of Care

Diagnostic Tests:

How will this test affect the management of the condition being evaluated?

Will this test possibly lead to more tests?

What are the risks to my health from this tests or follow-up tests?

What are the risks to my health from not having this test?

Treatments and Procedures:

What are the benefits of this treatment, medication, or procedure to my health?

Will it affect my quality of life?

Will it reduce my symptoms?

Will it help me live longer?

What are the possible side effects or complications from this treatment, medication, or procedure?

Do I need more time to consider?

Questions to ask before agreeing to undergo a test, treatment, or procedure to avoid unnecessary risks and costs. Answers to these questions should be clear and logical. If the answers leave doubts, a second opinion is warranted.

4) Website Table

A selection of websites that provide reliable information:

- The **National Library of Medicine** offers a large variety of information and resources on a broad range of medical subjects through http://www.nlm.nih.gov/medlineplus/.
- Healthfinder.gov provides current news, a health library, and much more, (also available in Spanish) is a **U.S. government** site that has current information on many areas of medical care.
- General health information is available from the **Mayo Clinic** at http://www.mayoclinic.org/.
- **Stanford University** offers a site to search the medical literature for articles through highwire.stanford.edu/lists/freeart.dtl.
- The **Cochrane Collaboration** is an international library dedicated to making up-to-date, evidence-based information about the effects of healthcare readily available worldwide at www.cochrane.org/.
- **The National Institute of Mental Health** provides information on mental disorders at www.nimh.nih.gov/.
- https://www.mskcc.org/cancer-care/treatments/symptom-management/integrative-medicine/herbs from the **Memorial Sloan-Kettering Cancer Center** provides evidence-based information on herbs and botanicals as alternative sources of medical treatments.
- Information on **alternative and complementary medicine**, including current research trials and other news, is available at from the National Institute of Health at https://nccih.nih.gov/from their National Center for Complimentary and Integrative Health.
- **The Centers for Disease Control and Prevention** provides travel health information as well as a wide variety of other information at http://www.cdc.gov/travel.
- **Immunization Action Coalition** provides immunization and vaccination information for all age groups at http://www. immunize.org/.

- You can search for current **clinical research studies** on many different conditions in the U.S at www.clinicaltrials.gov.
- **The American Heart Association** is a resource for cardiovascular disease; information at www.heart.org/HEARTORG/.
- **The National Cancer Institute** focuses on cancer types, treatments and clinical trials at www.cancer.gov.
- A virtual atlas of the human body can be found at http://www.ikonet.com/en/health/virtual-human-body/virtualhumanbody.php.
- A reliable web site sponsored by **Harvard University** information is http://www.health.harvard.edu/.
- The National Health Service from the UK has developed a web site to provide independent expert commentaries on topical medical matters reported in the international news media at http://www.nhs.uk/news/Pages/NewsIndex.aspx/.
- National Institute for Health Care Excellence (NICE) from the UK provides evidence-based guidance on medical conditions at nice.org.uk.

6) Advance Directives Tables

Uses and value of a Living Will

Provides a format to discuss specific situations and how you would want your patient advocate and healthcare providers to react to these.

Allows your patient advocate to understand your wishes and visualize being in the position of making healthcare decisions for you.

Allows your patient advocate to react to your wishes and choices, and to be clear that they can carry them out for you.

Periodic review of your living will with your patient advocate to clarify your wishes and current thinking is recommended.

Necessary attributes to the Patient Advocate you appoint

Patient Advocate:

Makes health care decisions for you when you are not capable.

The advocate should understand your wishes *and* your values.

The advocate should be willing and prepared to invoke your wishes if necessary.

Periodic discussions of these matters with your advocate assures that the advocate is clear and up to date on your thinking about your health care wishes and values.

The advocate must be available and accessible to make decisions on an hour to hour basis.

7) Living Will

This is the form from Michigan as an example of a Living Will document. (Reprinted with permission)

I, _____ am of sound mind, and I voluntarily make this declaration.

If I become terminally ill or permanently unconscious as determined by my doctor and at least one other doctor, and if I am unable to participate in decisions regarding my medical care, I intend this declaration to be honored as the expression of my legal right to authorize or refuse medical treatment.

My desires concerning medical treatment are—

_____
_____
_____
_____
_____
_____
_____
_____
_____
_____
_____
_____
_____
_____
_____
_____

My family, the medical facility, and any doctors, nurses and other medical personnel involved in my care shall have no civil or criminal liability for following my wishes as expressed in this declaration.

I may change my mind at any time by communicating in any manner that this declaration does not reflect my wishes.

Photostatic copies of this document, after it is signed and witnessed, shall have the same legal force as the original document.

I sign this document after careful consideration. I understand its meaning and I accept its consequences.

Dated: _____ Signed: _____
(Your signature)

_____

(Address)

STATEMENT OF WITNESSES

We sign below as witnesses. This declaration was signed in our presence. The declarant appears to be of sound mind, and to be making this designation voluntarily, without duress, fraud or undue influence.

_____   _____

(Print Name)   (Signature of Witness)

_____

(Address)

_____   _____

(Print Name)   (Signature of Witness)

_____

(Address)

8) DURABLE POWER OF ATTORNEY FOR HEALTH CARE

This is an example from Michigan of the Durable Power of Attorney form (reprinted with permission).

I, _____, am of sound mind and I voluntarily make this designation.

(Print or type your full name)

APPOINTMENT OF PATIENT ADVOCATE

I designate _____, my _____
    (Insert name of patient advocate) (Spouse, child, friend…)

living at _____
                (Address of patient advocate)
as my patient advocate. If my first choice cannot serve, I designate _____, my _____, living at
    (Name of successor patient advocate) (Spouse, child, friend…)

_____

_____
            (Address of successor patient advocate)
to serve as patient advocate.

My patient advocate or successor patient advocate must sign an acceptance before he or she can act. I have discussed this appointment with the individuals I have designated as patient advocate and successor patient advocate.

GENERAL POWERS

My patient advocate or successor patient advocate shall have power to make care, custody and medical treatment decisions for me if my attending physician and another physician or licensed psychologist determine I am unable to participate in medical treatment decisions.

In making decisions, my patient advocate shall try to follow my previously expressed wishes, whether I have stated them orally, in a living will, or in this designation.

My patient advocate has authority to consent to or refuse treatment on my behalf, to arrange medical and personal services for me, including admission to a hospital or nursing care facility, and to pay for such services with my funds.

My patient advocate shall have access to any of my medical records to which I have a right, immediately upon signing an Acceptance. This shall serve as a release under the Health Insurance Portability and Accountability Act.

Immediately upon signing an Acceptance, my patient advocate shall have access to my birth certificate and other legal documents needed to apply for Medicare, Medicaid, and other government programs.

POWER REGARDING LIFE-SUSTAINING TREATMENT
(OPTIONAL)

I expressly authorize my patient advocate to make decisions to withhold or withdraw treatment which would allow me to die, and I acknowledge such decisions could or would allow my death. My patient advocate can sign a do-not-resuscitate declaration for me. My patient advocate can refuse food and water administered to me through tubes.

(Sign your name if you wish to give your patient advocate this authority)

POWER REGARDING MENTAL HEALTH TREATMENT
(OPTIONAL)

I expressly authorize my patient advocate to make decisions concerning the following treatments if a physician and a mental health professional determine I cannot give informed consent for mental health care:

(check one or more consistent with your wishes)

- outpatient therapy

- my admission as a formal voluntary patient to a hospital to receive inpatient mental health services. I have the right to give three days notice of my intent to leave the hospital.

- my admission to a hospital to receive inpatient mental health services

- psychotropic medication

- electro-convulsive therapy (ECT)

I give up my right to have a revocation effective immediately. If I revoke my designation, the revocation is effective 30 days from the date I communicate my intent to revoke. Even if I choose this option, I still have the right to give three days notice of my intent to leave a hospital if I am a formal voluntary patient.

(Sign your name if you wish to give your patient advocate this authority)

POWER REGARDING ORGAN DONATION
(OPTIONAL)

I expressly authorize my patient advocate to make a gift of the following—

(check any that reflect your wishes)

- any needed organs or body parts for the purposes of transplantation, therapy, medical research or education

- only the following listed organs or body parts for the purposes of transplantation, therapy, medical research or education: _____

_____

- my entire body for anatomical study

- (optional) I wish my gift to go to—

_____

(Insert name of doctor, hospital, school, organ bank or individual)

The gift is effective upon my death. Unlike other powers I give to my patient advocate, this power remains after my death.

_____

(Sign your name if you wish to give your patient advocate this authority)

STATEMENT OF WISHES

My patient advocate has authority to make decisions in a wide variety of circumstances. In this document, I can express general wishes regarding conditions such as terminal illness, permanent unconsciousness, or other disability; specify particular types of treatment I do or not want in such circumstances; or I may state no wishes at all. If you have chosen to give your patient advocate power concerning mental health treatment, you can also include specific wishes about mental health treatment such as a preferred mental health professional, hospital or medication.

A. My wishes are as follows (you may attach more sheets of paper):

_____

_____

_____

_____

_____

_____

_____

_____

_____

or

I choose not to express any wishes in this document. This choice shall not be interpreted as limiting the power of my patient advocate to make any particular decision in any particular circumstance.

I may change my mind at any time by communicating in any manner that this designation does not reflect my wishes.

It is my intent no one involved in my care shall be liable for honoring my wishes as expressed in this designation or for following the directions of my patient advocate.

Photocopies of this document can be relied upon as though they were originals.

SIGNATURE

I sign this document voluntarily, and I understand its purpose.

Dated:_____

Signed:_____
(Your signature)

_____

_____
(Address)

STATEMENT REGARDING WITNESSES

I have chosen two adult witnesses who are not named in my will; who are not my spouse, parent, child, grandchild, brother or sister; who are not my physician or my patient advocate; who are not an employee of my life or health insurance company, an employee of a home for the aged where I reside, an employee of community mental health program providing me services or an employee at the health care facility where I am now.

STATEMENT AND SIGNATURE OF WITNESSES

We sign below as witnesses. This declaration was signed in our presence. The declarant appears to be of sound mind, and to be making this designation voluntarily, without duress, fraud or undue influence.

_____   _____
(Print Name)   (Signature of Witness)

_____
(Address)

_____   _____
(Print Name)   (Signature of Witness)

_____
(Address)

ACCEPTANCE BY PATIENT ADVOCATE

(1) This designation shall not become effective unless the patient is unable to participate in decisions regarding the patient's medical or mental health, as applicable. If this patient advocate designation includes the authority to make an anatomical gift as described in section 5506, the authority remains exercisable after the patient's death.

(2) A patient advocate shall not exercise powers concerning the patient's care, custody and medical or mental health treatment that the patient, if the patient were able to participate in the decision, could not have exercised in his or her own behalf.

(3) This designation cannot be used to make a medical treatment decision to withhold or withdraw treatment from a patient who is pregnant that would result in the pregnant patient's death.

(4) A patient advocate may make a decision to withhold or withdraw treatment which would allow a patient to die only if the patient has expressed in a clear and convincing manner that the patient advocate is authorized to make such a decision, and that the patient acknowledges that such a decision could or would allow the patient's death.

(5) A patient advocate shall not receive compensation for the performance of his or her authority, rights, and responsibilities, but a patient advocate may be reimbursed for actual and necessary expenses incurred in the performance of his or her authority, rights, and responsibilities.

(6) A patient advocate shall act in accordance with the standards of care applicable to fiduciaries when acting for the patient and shall act consistent with the patient's best interests. The known desires of the patient expressed or evidenced while the patient is able to participate in medical or mental heath treatment decisions are presumed to be in the patient's best interests.

(7) A patient may revoke his or her designation at any time or in any manner sufficient to communicate an intent to revoke.

(8) A patient may waive his or her right to revoke the patient advocate designation as to the power to make mental health treatment decisions, and if such waiver is made, his or her ability to revoke as to certain treatment will be delayed for 30 days after the patient communicates his or her intent to revoke.

(9) A patient advocate may revoke his or her acceptance to the designation at any time and in any manner sufficient to communicate an intent to revoke.

(10) A patient admitted to a health facility or agency has the rights enumerated in Section 20201 of the Public Health Code, Act No. 368 of the Public Acts of 1978, Being Section 333.20201 of the Michigan Compiled Laws.

I, _____, understand the above
                    (Name of patient advocate)
conditions and I accept the designation as patient advocate or successor
patient advocate for _____, who signed a
                              (Name of patient)
durable power of attorney for health care on the following date:_____.

Dated:_____

Signed:_____
        (Signature of patient advocate or successor patient advocate)

The following is a Do Not Resuscitate form from Michigan (reprinted with permission).

9) DO-NOT-RESUSCITATE ORDER

I have discussed my health status with my physician, _____. I request that in the event my heart and breathing should stop, no person shall attempt to resuscitate me.
This order is effective until it is revoked by me.
Being of sound mind, I voluntarily execute this order, and I understand its full import.

_____   _____
(Declarant's signature)   (Date)

_____
          (Type or print declarant's full name)

_____
(Signature of person who signed for declarant, if applicable)

                                                          _____
                                                          (Date)

_____
(Type or print full name)

_____   _____
(Physician's signature)   (Date)

_____
          (Type or print physician's full name)

ATTESTATION OF WITNESSES

The individual who has executed this order appears to be of sound mind, and under no duress, fraud, or undue influence. Upon executing this order, the individual has (has not) received an identification bracelet.

(Witness signature)   (Date)

(Witness signature)   (Date)

(Type or print witness's name)   (Type or print witness's name)

THIS FORM WAS PREPARED PURSUANT TO, AND IN COMPLIANCE WITH, THE MICHIGAN DO-NOT-RESUSCITATE PROCEDURE ACT

References

Preface
Daniel Kahneman
Thinking Fast and Slow
Farrar, Straus, and Giroux, 2011

Prologue

Barry MJ, Kaufman DS, and Wu CL
Case 15-2008—A 55-Year-Old Man with an Elevated Prostate-Specific Antigen Level and Early-Stage Prostate Cancer
N Engl J Med; 2008; 358:2161-2168

Bill-Axelson A., Holmberg L., Ruutu M., Häggman M., Andersson S.-O., Bratell S., Spångberg A., Busch C., Nordling S., Garmo H., Palmgren J., Adami H.-O., Norlén B. J., Johansson J.-E., the Scandinavian Prostate Cancer Group Study No. 4
Radical Prostatectomy versus Watchful Waiting in Early Prostate Cancer
N Engl J Med; May 12, 2005; 352:1977-1984,

Johansson JE, Andren O, Andersson SO, et al
Natural history of early, localized prostate cancer.
JAMA; 2004; 291:2713-2719.

Zietman AL, Thakral H, Wilson L, Schellhammer P
Conservative Management of Prostate Cancer in the Prostate Specific Antigen Era: The Incidence and Time course of Subsequent Therapy
Journal of Urology; 2001; 166: 1702-1706.

Chapter 1: Exercising Autonomy in Medical Decision Making

Epstein RM, Alper BS, Quill TE
Communicating Evidence for Participatory Decision Making
JAMA; May 19, 2004; 291: 2359-2366

Ford S; Schofield T; Hope T
What are the Ingredients for a Successful Evidence Based Patient Choice Consult?
Social Science and Medicine; 2003; 56 589-598.

Horton, Richard
The Lessons of MMR
The Lancet; 6 March 2004; 363(9411): 747-749

Humink, Myriam and Grasziou, Paul
Decision Making in Health and Medicine
Cambridge University Press, 2001

Kennedy ADM, Sculpher MSJ, Coulter A, Dwyer N, Rees M, Abrams KR, Horsley S, Cowley; D, Kidson C, Kirwin D, Naish C, Stirrat G
Effects of Decision Aids for Menorrhagia on Treatment Choices, Health Outcomes, and Costs: A Randomized Controlled Trial
JAMA; Dec 2002; 288: 2701-2708

Offit, Paul A., MD
Autism's False Prophets: Bad Science, Risky Medicine, and the Search for a Cure.
Columbia Univ. Press, Sept. 2008

Whelan T, Sawka C, Levine M, Gafni A, Reyno L, Willan A, Julian J, Dent S, Abu-Zahra H, Chouinard E, Tozer R, Pritchard K, and Bodendorfer I
Helping Patients Make Informed Choices: A Randomized Trial of a Decision Aid for Adjuvant Chemotherapy in Lymph Node-

Negative Breast Cancer
J Natl Cancer Inst; Apr 2003; 95: 581.

Chapter 2: Perceptions of Risk

Bogardus Jr ST, Holmboe E,. Jekel JF
Perils, Pitfalls, and Possibilities in Talking About Medical Risk
JAMA; Mar 1999; 281: 1037-1041

Epstein RM, Alper BS, Quill TE
Communicating Evidence for Participatory Decision Making
JAMA; May 19, 2004; 291: 2359-2366

Ford S; Schofield T; Hope T
What are the Ingredients for a Successful Evidence Based Patient Choice Consult?
Social Science and Medicine; 2003; 56 589-598.

Humink, Myriam and Grasziou, Paul
Decision Making in Health and Medicine
Cambridge University Press, 2001

Katz JN
Patient Preferences and Health Disparities
JAMA; Sep 2001; 286: 1506-1509

McNutt RA
Shared Medical Decision Making: Problems, Process, Progress
JAMA; November 24, 2004; 292: 2516-2518

Chapter 3: Emotions and Bias

Brinkman P, Coates D
Lottery Winners and Accident Victims: is Happiness Relative?
J Pers Soc Psychol; 1978; 36: 917-927

Epstein RM, Alper BS, Quill TE
Communicating Evidence for Participatory Decision Making
JAMA; May 19, 2004; 291: 2359-2366

Ford S; Schofield T; Hope T
What are the Ingredients for a Successful Evidence Based Patient Choice Consult?
Social Science and Medicine, 2003; 56 589-598

Humink, Myriam and Grasziou, Paul
Decision Making in Health and Medicine
Cambridge University Press, 2001

Katz RN
Patient Preferences and Health Disparities
JAMA; Sep 2001; 286: 1506-1509

McNutt RA
Shared Medical Decision Making: Problems, Process, Progress
JAMA; November 24, 2004; 292: 2516-2518

Redelmeier DA, Rozin P, Kahneman D
Understanding Patients' Decisions. Cognitive and Emotional Perspectives
JAMA; Jul 1993; 270: 72-76

Chapter 4: Going to the Doctor

Ad Hoc Committee on Health Literacy for the Council on Scientific Affairs, American Medical Association
Health Literacy: Report of the Council on Scientific Affairs
JAMA; Feb 1999; 281: 552-557

Gazmararian JA, Baker DW, Williams MV, Parker RM, Scott TL, Green DC, Fehrenbach SN, Ren J, Koplan JP

Health Literacy Among Medicare Enrollees in a Managed Care Organization
JAMA; Feb 1999; 281: 545-551

Kravitz RL R. Hays D, Sherbourne CD, DiMatteo MR, Rogers WH, Ordway L, Greenfield S
Recall of recommendations and adherence to advice among patients with chronic medical conditions
Archives of Internal Medicine; Aug 1993; 153: 1869-1878.

Lasker RD and Marquis MS
The Intensity of Physicians' Work in Patient Visits—Implications for the Coding of Patient Evaluation and Management Services
N Engl J Med; Jul 1999; 341: 337-341

Marvel MK, Epstein RM, Flowers K, Beckman HB
Soliciting the Patient's Agenda: Have We Improved?
JAMA; Jan 1999; 281: 283-287.

Mechanic D., McAlpine D. D., Rosenthal M.
Are Patient's Office Visits With Physicians Getting Shorter?
N Engl J Med; Jan 18, 2001; 344:198-204,

Chapter 5: More Care may not be Better Care

Anderson GF, Chalkidou K
Spending on Medical Care: More Is Better?
JAMA; 2008; 299(20):2444-2445

Bangalore s. Maron DJ, Hochman JS,
Evidence-Baed Management of Stable Ischemic Heart Disease
JAMA; 2015; 314: 1917-1918

Brownlee S
The Overtreated American
The Atlantic Monthly; Jan/Feb 2003

Chassin MR, Galvin RW and the National Roundtable on Health Care Quality
The Urgent Need to Improve Health Care Quality
Institute of Medicine National Roundtable on Health Care Quality
JAMA; 1998; 280:1000-1005.

Cram P, Rosenthal GE
Physician-Owned Specialty Hospitals and Coronary Revascularization Utilization: Too Much of a Good Thing?
JAMA; 2007; 297:998-999.

Deyo RA and Patrick DL
Hope or Hype
AMACOM press, 2005

Fisher ES
Medical Care—Is More Always Better?
N Engl J Med; Oct 23, 2003; 349:1665-1667,

Fisher ES, Welch HG
Avoiding the Unintended Consequences of Growth in Medical Care: How Might More Be Worse?
JAMA; 1999; 281:446-453.

Hadler NM
Worried Sick
The University of North Carolina Press, Chapel Hill, 2008

Mitka, Mike
Less May be More When Managing Patients With Severe Chronic Illness
JAMA; July 12, 2006; 296:2,

Redberg Rita, Walsh Judith
Pay Now, Benefits May Follow—The Case of Cardiac Computed Tomographic Angiography
N Engl J Med; 2008; 359: 2309-2311

Seematter-Bagnoud L, Vader J-P, Wietlisbach V, Froehlich F, Gonvers J-J, and
Burnand B
Overuse and Underuse of Diagnostic Upper Gastrointestinal Endoscopy in Various Clinical Settings
Int. J. Qual. Health Care; Aug 1999; 11: 301-308.

Shekelle PG, Kahan JP, Bernstein SJ, Leape LL, Kamberg CJ, Park RE
The Reproducibility of a Method to Identify the Overuse and Underuse of Medical Procedures
N Engl J Med.; Jun 1998; 338: 1888-1895.

Stone J. H.
Incidentalomas—Clinical Correlation and Translational Science Required
N Engl J Med; Jun 29, 2006; 354:2748-2749,

Wennberg JE, ed.
The Dartmouth atlas of health care in the United States/2006
Chicago: American Hospital Publishing

Wennberg J E, Gittelsohn A
Small area variations in health care delivery
Science; 1973; 182:1102-1108

Chapter 6: **Thieves of Autonomy**

Cassell EJ, M.D
Consent or Obedience? Power and Authority in Medicine.
New England Journal of Medicine; 352; 4: 328-330

Cassell EJ, Leon AC, Kaufman SG
Preliminary Evidence of Impaired Thinking in Sick Patients.
Annals of Internal Medicine; 2001; 134 1120-1123

Jadad AR, Rizo CA, Enkin MW
I am a good patient, believe it or not
BMJ; 2003; 326:1293-1295

Chapter 7: Aging and Health Care Choices

Boult C, Boult LB, et. Al.
**A Randomized Clinical Trial of Outpatient Geriatric Evaluation
and Management**
Journal of the American Geriatric Society; 49 (2001), p.351

Christakis Na, Lamont EB
**Extent and determinants of error in doctors' prognoses in
terminally ill patients: prospective cohort study**
British Medical Journal; 320 (2000), p.469

Connor SR, Pyenson B, et. Al.
**Comparing Hospice and Nonhospice Patient Survival Among
Patients Who Die Within a Three-Year Window**
Journal of Pain and Symptom Management; 33 (2007), p.238

Emanuel Ezekiel J
Why I Hope to Die at 75
Atlantic; October 2014; http://www.theatlantic.com/magazine/
archive/2014/10/why-i-hope-to-die-at-75/379329/

Gawande Atul
Being Mortal
Metropolitan Books/Henry Holt; 2014

Gordon EJ and Daugherty CK
**"Hitting you over the head": Oncologists' disclosure of prognosis
to advanced cancer patients**
Bioethics; 17 (2003), p.142

McCullough Dennis
My Mother, Your Mother
Harper; 2008

Spettell CM, Rawlins WS, et. Al.
A Comprehensive Case Management Program to Improve Palliative Care
Journal of Palliative Medicine; 12 (2009), p.827

Temel JS, Greer JA, et. Al.
Early Palliative Care for Patients with Metastatic Non-Small-Cell Lung Cancer
New Eng J of Med; 363 (2010), p.733

Chapter 8: **Choices as the End of Life Approaches**

American Medical Association Code of Medical Ethics, 2016 Revision
Chapter 5: Opinions on Caring for Patients at the End of Life
http://www.ama-assn.org/ama/pub/physician-resources/medical-ethics/code-medical-ethics.page, accessed July 15, 2016.

Eddy DM,
A Conversation with My Mother
JAMA; 272 (1994), p.179

Fischer SM, Beckman D, Bailey FA
Family Assessment of Quality of Care In the Last Month of Life
JAMA Internal Medicine; Published online June 26. 2016; http://archinte.jamanetwork.com/article.aspx?articleID=2529495

Ganzini L, Goy ER, et. Al;
Nurses' Experience with Hospice Patients who Refuse Food and Fluids to Hasten Death
New England Journal of Medicine; 349, July 24, 2003: 359-365

Gross J **What an End-of-Life Adviser Could Have Told Me New York Times,** *The New Old Age;* December 15, 2008

Rietjens JA, van Delden J, van der Heide A, Vrakking AM **Terminal Sedation and Euthanasia: A Comparison of Clinical Practices** **Arch Intern Med;** 2006; 166: 749-753

Sacks Oliver **My Own Life** **New York Times,** *The Opinion Pages;* February 19, 2015

Final Certainty **The Economist;** June 27, 2015

Chapter 9: Advance Directives

Evelyn, MH and Alfonso, AM **Pre Arrest Predictors of Failure to Survive after In-hospital Cardiopulmonary Resuscitation** **Family Practice;** 2011; 28: 505-515

O'Reilly KB **AMA Meeting: AMA OKs Palliative Sedation for Terminally Ill** **American Medical News;** July 7, 2008

Quill TE **Initiating End-of-Life Discussions with Seriously Ill Patients: Addressing the "Elephant in the Room"** **JAMA;** Nov 2000; 284: 2502-2507

Schneider CE and Fagerlin A **The Death of the Living Will** **Hasting Center Reports;** Volume 34; March-April 2004:30-42

Silveira MJ, Kim S, Langa KM **Advance Directives and Outcomes of Surrogate Decision Making**

Before Death
New England Journal of Medicine; 2010; 362: 1211-1218

Teno JM, Licks S, Lynn J
Do advance directives provide instructions that direct care? SUPPORT Investigators. Study to Understand Prognoses and Preferences for Outcomes and Risks of Treatment.
J Am Geriatr Soc; Apr 1, 1997; 45(4): 508-12

Teno J, Lynn J, Wenger N
Advance directives for seriously ill hospitalized patients: effectiveness with the patient self-determination act and the SUPPORT intervention. SUPPORT Investigators. Study to Understand Prognoses and Preferences for Outcomes and Risks of Treatment.
J Am Geriatr Soc; Apr 1, 1997; 45(4): 500-7

Teno JM, Stevens M, Spernak S, Lynn J
Role of Written Advance Directives in Decision Making Insights from Qualitative and Quantitative Data
Journal of the American Geriatric Soc; 1997:439-46

Tierney WM, Dexter PR, Gramelspacher GP, Perkins AJ, Zhou X-H, Wolinsky FD
The Effect of Discussions about Advance Directives on Patients' Satisfaction with Primary Care
J Gen Intern Med; 2001; 16:32-40

Tsevat J, Dawson NV, Wu AW, Lynn J,. Soukup JR, Cook EF, Vidaillet H, Phillips RS, for the HELP Investigators
Health Values of Hospitalized Patients 80 Years or Older
JAMA; Feb 1998; 279: 371.

The SUPPORT Principal Investigators
A controlled trial to improve care for seriously ill hospitalized adults: the Study to Understand Prognoses and Preferences for Outcomes and Risks of Treatments (SUPPORT).
JAMA; 1995; 274:1591-1598

Wright AA, Zhang B, et. Al.
Associations Between End-Of-Life Discussions, Patient Mental Health Near Death, and Caregiver Bereavement
JAMA; 2008; 300: 1665-1673

Chapter 10: Gathering Information

Bartlett C, Sterne J, and Egger M
What is newsworthy? Longitudinal study of the reporting of medical research in two British newspapers
BMJ; Jul 2002; 325: 81

Bell CM, Urbach DR, Ray, JG, Bayoumi A, Rosen AB, Greenberg D, Neumann PJ
Bias in published cost effectiveness studies: systematic review
BMJ; 2006; 332:699-703.

Coiera E
Information Economics and the Internet
Journal of the American Medical Informatics Association; 2000: 7:215-221

Dentzer, Susan
Communicating Medical News—Pitfalls of Health Care Journalism
New England Journal of Medicine; Jan 1, 2009: 360: 1-3

Dickersin K
The existence of publication bias and risk factors for its occurrence
JAMA; 1990; 263:1385-1389

Epstein JI, Walsh PC, Sanfilippo F
Clinical and cost impact of second-opinion pathology. Review of prostate biopsies prior to radical prostatectomy.
Am J Surg Pathol; 1996; 20: 851-7

Eysenbach G, Powell J, Kuss O, Sa E-R
Empirical Studies Assessing the Quality of Health Information for Consumers on the World Wide Web: A Systematic Review
JAMA; May 2002; 287: 2691-2700

Graboys TB. Biegelsen B. Lampert S. Blatt CM. Lown B.
Results of a second-opinion trial among patients recommended for coronary angiography
JAMA; 1992; 268: 2537-40

Haynes RB, Cotoi C, Holland J, Walters L, Wilczynski N, Jedraszewski D, McKinlay J, Parrish R,McKibbon KA, for the McMaster Premium Literature Service (PLUS) Project
Second-Order Peer Review of the Medical Literature for Clinical Practitioners
JAMA; April 19, 2006; 295: 1801-1808

Liebeskind DS, Kidwell CS, Sayre JW, Saver JL.
Evidence of Publication Bias in Reporting Acute Stroke Clinical Trials.
Neurology; 2006 Sep 26; 67(6):973-9

Liss, R.
Publication Bias in the Pulmonary/allergy Literature: Effect of Pharmaceutical Company Sponsorship.
Isr Med Assoc J; Jul 8, 2006 (7):451-4

Markoff, John
Microsoft Examines Causes of "Cyberchondria"
New York Times, *Health Section;* November 24, 2008

Ridker PM, Torres J
Reported Outcomes in Major Cardiovascular Clinical Trials Funded by For-Profit and Not-for-Profit Organizations: 2000-2005
JAMA; 2006; 295:2270-2274

Schwartz LM, Woloshin S
The Media Matter: A Call for Straightforward Medical Reporting
Annals of Internal Medicine; February 3, 2004; 140(3): 226-228

Schwartz LM, Woloshin S, Baczek L
Media Coverage of Scientific Meetings
Too Much, Too Soon?
JAMA; 2002; 287:2859-2863.

Woloshin S, and Schwartz LM
What's the Rush? The Dissemination and Adoption of Preliminary Research Results
J National Cancer Inst; 2006; 98:372-373

Chapter 11: Participation in Clinical Research

Agrawal M, Grady C, Fairclough DL, Meropol NJ, Maynard K, and Emanuel EJ **Patients' Decision-Making Process Regarding Participation in Phase I Oncology Research**
J. Clinical Oncology; Sep 2006; 24: 4479-4484.

Horstmann E, McCabe M S, Grochow L, Yamamoto S, Rubinstein L, Budd T, Shoemaker D, Emanuel E J, Grady C
Risks and Benefits of Phase 1 Oncology Trials, 1991 through 2002
N Engl J Med; Mar 3, 2005; 352:895-904

Kurzrock R, Benjamin R S
Risks and Benefits of Phase 1 Oncology Trials, Revisited
N Engl J Med; 2005; Mar 3, 2005:930-932

Lidz GW, Applebaum PS
The Therapeutic Misconception
Medical Care; 2002; 40: Vol. 9, Supplement V53-63

Miller FG, Rosentstein DL
The Therapeutic Orientation to Clinical Trials
N Engl J Med; April 3, 2003; 348: 1383-1386,

Peppercorn J M, Weeks J C, Cook E F, Steven J
Comparison of outcomes in cancer patients treated within and outside clinical trials: conceptual framework and structured review
Lancet; 2004; 363:263-270

Wendler D, Krohmal B, Emanuel EJ, Grady C, for the ESPRIT Group
Why Patients Continue to Participate in Clinical Research
Arch Intern Med; 2008; 168(12):1294-1299.

Chapter 12: Experience and Volume Matters

Bartels DB, Wypij D, Wenzlaff P, Dammann O, Poets CF
Hospital Volume and Neonatal Mortality among Very Low Birth Weight Infants
Pediatrics; Vol. 117 No. 6 June 2006, pp. 2206-2214 (doi:10.1542/peds.2005-1624)

Choudhry NK, Fletcher RH, and Soumerai SB
Systematic Review: The Relationship between Clinical Experience and Quality of Health Care
Ann Intern Med; Feb 2005; 142: 260-273

Fender D, van der Meulen JHP, and Gregg PJ
Relationship between outcome and annual surgical experience for the Charnley total hip replacement
RESULTS FROM A REGIONAL HIP REGISTER
J Bone Joint Surg Br; Mar 2003; 85-B: 187-190

Finlayson SRG
Delivering Quality to Patients
JAMA; 2006; 296:2026-2027

Halm EA, Lee C, and Chassin MR
Is Volume Related to Outcome in Health Care? A Systematic Review and Methodologic Critique of the Literature
Ann Intern Med; Sep 2002; 137: 511-520.

Hammond JW, Queale WS, Kim TK, McFarland EG
Surgeon Experience and Clinical and Economic Outcomes for Shoulder Arthroplasty
The Journal of Bone and Joint Surgery (American*)*; 2003; 85:2318-2324

Khan K, Campbell A, Wallington T, Gardam M
The impact of Physician Training and Experience on the Survival of Patients with Active Tuberculosis.
Can Med Assoc J; 2006; 175: 749-753

Kitahata M M, Koepsell T D, Deyo R A, Maxwell C L, Dodge W T, Wagner E H **Physicians' Experience with the Acquired Immunodeficiency Syndrome as a Factor in Patients' Survival**
N Engl J Med; Mar 14, 1996; 334:701-707,

Laffel G., Barnett A I, Finkelstein., Kaye M P
The Relation Between Experience and Outcome in Heart Transplantation
N Engl J Med; Oct 22, 1992; 327:1220-1225

Meltzer D, Manning WG, Morrison J, Shah MN, Sin L, Guth T, Levinson W
Effects of Physician Experience on Costs and Outcomes on an Academic General Medicine Service: Results of a Trial of Hospitalists
Annals of Internal Medicine; 3 December 2002: 137 (11): 866-874

O'Brien SM, DeLong ER, Peterson ED
Impact of Case Volume on Hospital Performance Assessment
Arch Intern Med*;* 2008; 168(12):1277-1284.

Reznick RK and MacRae H
Medical Education: Teaching Surgical Skills—Changes in the Wind
New England Journal of Medicine; Volume 35 December 21, 2006

Personal Observations 4

Bull Margaret J, and McShane Ruth E
Needs and Supports for Family Caregivers of Chronically Ill Elders
Home Health Care Management Practice, Feb 2002; 14: 92-98

Cammeron, J.L. and the Canadian Critical Care Trials Group
One-Year Outcomes in Caregivers of Critically Ill Patients
New England Journal of Medicine; Volume 374, May 12, 2016

Grov EK, Dahl AA, Moum T, and Fosså SD
Anxiety, depression, and quality of life in caregivers of patients with cancer in late palliative phase
Annals of Oncoclogy; Jul 2005; 16: 1185-1191.

Hauser Winfried, Bernardy Kathrin, Uceyler Nurcan, and Sommer, Claudia
Treatment of Fibromyalgia Syndrome with Antidepressants
JAMA; Jan 14, 2009; 301(2): 198-209

Index

A

Adherence,...84
Attribution bias,..48
Autonomy,........................11, 13, 21, 29, 82, 91, 93,123,156,187-188
Availability bias,...46, 126

B

Beneficence,..21
Blind randomized trial,...156

C

Clinical research,...142, 153-159
Compliance,..84
Confirmation bias,...44-45
Conflicts of interest,...19, 74, 187-188
Consumerism,..57
CPR (cardio-pulmonary resuscitation),.......................................132
Cultural competence,...109-110, 189-190
Cyberchondria,..143

D

Dartmouth Atlas of Health Care,...70, 102
Death with Dignity Laws,...115, 118-120
Disgust,..52-53
Doctrine of double effect,...119
DNR or Do Not Resuscitate,...123, 131-132
Durable Power of Attorney for Health Care,....123, 129-131, 134, 214

E

Emanuel, Ezekiel,...93, 96-98

F

False negative,..76
False positive,..76-77
File drawer problem,..156
Framing,..39-40

G

Gawande, Atul,...93-96
Geriatrics,..91

H

Hickam's Dictum,..49
Health section of newspapers,..149
Heuristics,...31, 186
Hospice,..117-114

I

Incentives for More Care,...73, 111
Incidentaloma,...75-76
Informed choice,...11, 29, 137
Informed consent,...29
Institutional Review Board,...157
Internet,...32, 139-143
Irrational reactions,..52-53

J

J-shaped curve,...42, 43
Justice,..21

K

Kahneman, Daniel,..14

L

Living will,..123, 128-129, 211

M

McCullough, Dennis,..93, 101-102
Medical ethics,..21, 29, 119, 157,187

Medicalese,...147, 200
Medical information,..............................32, 13, 139-152, 209-210
Medical journals,...146-148
Medical terminology,..147, 200
Medical text books,..146-148
Miscalibration,...37

N
News media,...148-149
Non-maleficence,...21

O
Occam's Razor,...49
Overuse of health care,..70

P
Palliative care,..114-115
Patient-advocate,...129-130, 134, 211
Patient controlled death,..118-120
Physician-assisted death,...118-119
Predicting future feelings,...45-46
Preference for the status quo,...49-52, 186
Primary care provider,.......................................14, 160, 186-193
Pseudodisease,...75
Pseudoscience,...150-152
Publication bias,..156

R
Redirection,..60-61, 105
Reference point,...51-52
Regret,..39
Risk,..36
Risk calculator,..201-205

S
Sacks, Oliver,..109
Second opinion,..80, 143-146, 192

Slow medicine,..93, 101-104
Slow planet,..101
Sound bite,..126
Specialty institutions,..161
Support,..64, 106, 179-182
Surrogate markers,..173-175

T
Terminal sedation,..115-118
Tertiary care centers,..167
Therapeutic misconception,..155

V
Voluntarily stopping eating and drinking (VSED),..................120-122

W
Worry,..53-54

Z
Zero risk,..37